PainEDU.org Manual
A POCKET GUIDE TO PAIN MANAGEMENT

A Companion to www.PainEDU.org

Kevin L. Zacharoff, M.D.
Lynette Menefee Pujol, Ph.D.
Evelyn Corsini, M.S.W.

Copyright 2010, Inflexxion®, Inc. All rights reserved
320 Needham Street, Suite 100
Newton, MA 02464

Produced for Inflexxion®, Inc. by:
Kevin L. Zacharoff, M.D.
Lynette Menefee Pujol, Ph.D.
Evelyn Corsini, M.S.W.

Reviewed by:
Robert Jamison, Ph.D.
Pain Management Center
Brigham & Women's Hospital
Boston, MA

Acknowledgment
The authors would like to acknowledge with deep appreciation and
gratitude, the work of Pravin Pant. This project only came to be
successfully completed through Pravin's perseverance and diligence
with respect to coordination and fact-checking at every level.

ISBN: 978-0-9740093-5-3

Supported through an educational grant from Endo Pharmaceuticals.

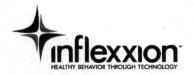

CONTENTS

Foreword

This manual is intended to serve as a valuable and informative pocket reference for those health care providers and health care students who are not experts in the field, but who are or will be faced daily with the management of patients with pain. We offer this guide as a resource to them as they inevitably encounter this common and difficult problem that presents in many forms.

We were motivated to develop the 4th edition by many things that have taken place since the 3rd edition. First, we have included all of the updates to the Manual that have been written for **www.PainEDU.org** since that printing. Second, new and significant events have taken place within the field of chronic pain management, including the release of a set of chronic opioid guidelines for the treatment of chronic noncancer pain, jointly developed by the American Pain Society and the American Academy of Pain Management. Finally, and most important, the response to the last edition was so overwhelmingly positive that it gave us the impetus to make it even better by listening to what registered users of PainEDU told us they would like to see covered in this text, and on the web site.

Despite the progress made in the field of pain management since the last edition, it is clear that the educational deficits in this important area still overshadow the advances. We consider this text to be a thoughtful, living, breathing document to help serve that need. We hope that it will be a handy tool to guide health care providers in the right direction toward the assessment, diagnosis, and appropriate treatment of common painful conditions.

As with past editions, although it is difficult to cover all conditions and details in a small text, we feel confident that this manual, in conjunction with its companion web site, ***www.PainEDU.org***, will continue to be an invaluable part of your quick-reference library for treating the common painful conditions affecting your patients' lives.

Kevin L. Zacharoff, M.D.
Lynette Menefee Pujol, Ph.D.
Evelyn Corsini, M.S.W.

I.

Basic Principles of Pain Management

BASICS OF PAIN TREATMENT

> "Cure sometimes, treat often, comfort always."
> —Hippocrates

Pain is a phenomenon that all people encounter at some point in their lives. Both a sensory and an emotional experience, pain is defined as being an unpleasant experience associated with actual or potential tissue damage. Pain, in both its acute and chronic manifestations, can commandeer a patient's body and mind. When improperly managed, pain can lead to decreased productivity and diminished quality of life.[1] The consequences of inadequate attention to pain reach into the professional, family, sexual, and vocational realms.

Although in many situations pain may not be curable, it is a treatable condition. As the science of pain continues to unravel the mystery of its mechanisms, health care providers have an increasingly large arsenal of tools to deploy against pain. There are new clinically accepted methods and guidelines for assessing and treating pain in adult, pediatric, and elderly populations. Each measure is calibrated to elicit the most accurate self-report from patients of certain age groups and levels of cognitive ability. In addition, a review of a patient's medical history and a thorough physical and neurologic examination can be useful tools in qualifying and quantifying pain.[2]

Using these measurement tools, a health care provider is empowered to treat pain with pharmacologic, nonpharmacologic, and psychological remedies. Treatment should be tailored to the type of pain, the location of the pain, its duration, and its intensity. Other considerations include, but are not limited to, the patient's medical history and previous reactions to particular drugs. Assessment of the psychological and social consequences of pain is an important part of tailoring treatment. Multimodal treatment strategies are often necessary to achieve success. Any pain treatment needs to be fine-tuned to a patient's particular needs. There is almost invariably a trial-and-error period while the regimen is adjusted. It is also essential that the patient and his or her family understand the limitations of pain management.

Modern society has high expectations for health care, and it is important to communicate that complete relief from pain is frequently not possible. Special considerations apply in cases of young patients, those who are cognitively impaired, those with psychiatric comorbidities, and patients at the end of life. In managing pain, the emphasis should be on effectively minimizing discomfort and maximizing function, while attending to its underlying cause.

When treating pain, regardless of the modalities used, some basic "pearls of wisdom" are worth keeping in mind (Table 1.1).

■ **Table 1.1**
  Basics of Pain Treatment

Analgesia should be integrated into a comprehensive patient evaluation and management plan.
The emotional and cognitive aspects of pain must be recognized and treated.
There is no reliable way to objectively measure pain.
Pain is most often undertreated, not over-treated.
Pain control must be individualized.
Anticipate rather than react to pain.
Whenever possible, let the patient control his or her own pain.
Pain control is often best achieved by rational polypharmacy.
Pain control often requires a multidisciplinary, team approach.

Adapted from Ducharme J. Acute pain and pain control: state of the art. *Ann EmergMed 2000;35:592–603.*

KEY COMPONENTS OF A
LOGICAL APPROACH TO MANAGING PAIN

Despite the fact that principles and tools exist for assessment and treatment of pain today, barriers exist that may hinder successful outcomes. Improved education about appropriate assessment and treatment of pain will, it is hoped, someday conquer some of these barriers and the myths they promote. Certainly, an important part of the process of effectively treating pain is to take a logical approach towards assessment and management. Here is a potential model of this kind of approach:

- *A detailed history and physical*   It is imperative for this critical step not only to fact find, but also to begin cementing a relationship that has the potential to make, or break, the successful treatment of pain. The clinician needs to establish the hallmark of an effective dialogue, trust and compassion for the patient's pain. This step also provides the opportunity for the clinician to listen and understand how to explore the impact of pain on the patient's life.

- *Any appropriate testing that can facilitate diagnosis*   There may or may not be any testing needed, depending on the signs and symptoms. A clinician may feel that the history and chief complaint point towards the diagnosis of migraine headache for example, and opt to treat with first-line therapy. On the other hand, for the patient presenting with low back pain of sudden onset and acute nature, the clinician may opt to order radiologic tests of the spine before intervening.

- *Establishment of realistic and desired common goals of further treatment and/or evaluation*   This would be the point where effective evaluation and treatment start to take a unique path. **It is critical for the clinician to understand what the patient is looking for in terms of successful treatment, regardless of the painful condition.** In some situations, the diagnostic answers might be clear, as in headaches, but the impact on the patient's life, quality of life, and ability to perform activities of daily living, must be identified, documented, and constantly revisited along the continuum of care.

■ ***Formulation of a treatment plan***   When treating pain, the clinician and the patient need to act as a team to identify measurable, beneficial hallmarks of therapy. The point of this is valuable in many ways; the most significant being the ability to measure success or failure. All parties should understand what those measures are, and what steps will be taken in the event success is not achieved at one point or another. If the patient understands what the alternative plans are up front, and that there indeed *are* alternative plans, they may be much more inclined to be more patient with therapeutic trials. This is also the time when the health care provider can detail what everyone's responsibilities are, from all perspectives, with respect to use of opioids or other controlled substances. This might be treatment agreements, periodic testing, and other risk management strategies.

■ ***Flexibility in modification of treatment based on periodic assessment and patient questioning***   A patient may become unstable in their pain treatment (i.e., experience periods of breakthrough pain) and require add-on therapy for a short period of time, or even rotation to a different form of drug or modality. Periodic reassessment is necessary to monitor progress, regression, patient compliance, and even exit strategies when opioids are employed.

■ ***Referral to a pain specialist***   The point at which a primary care clinician may opt to refer the patient to a specialist for treatment will vary based on experience, expertise, and comfort level with the medications and modalities necessary for treatment. A specialist may be able to use a more technically complex approach to pain management by attempting to modify the mechanism responsible for the pain. This might be beyond the scope of a primary care provider. The most successful dynamic between the primary care clinician and the pain specialist is when a treatment plan is formulated and implemented by the consultant, and information is communicated between the two clinicians.

As we look back at 2000 – 2010, which was designated the "Decade of Pain Control and Research" by the U.S. Congress[3], awareness has increased, attention to assessment has improved, but efficacy of treatment may be lagging behind. The health care system still lacks clearly articulated primary care practice standards for pain management, taking into consideration that most chronic pain patients present to their primary care providers for treatment. Other than the Joint Commission's institutional standards, there is a noticeable absence of accountability and competency for adequate assessment and management of pain. The growth of managed care has also led to fragmentation and lack of communication among clinicians, leading to less coordination of care. Financial barriers and lack of access to health care, ultimately lead to a lower level of care.

■ **Table 1.2**
Common Myths about Pain

Children do not feel pain to the same degree as adults.
It is not possible to adequately measure pain in cognitively impaired patients.
Physical manifestations of pain are more important than self-report measurements.
Pain does not exist in the absence of detectable tissue damage.
Pain without an obvious source is usually psychogenic.
The same stimulus produces the same degree of pain in all individuals.
Analgesic therapy should not be started until the cause of pain is established.
Noncancer pain is not as severe as cancer pain.
Knowledgeable patients have a higher incidence of drug diversion.
Use of opioids causes all patients to become addicted to them.
Aggressive pain management is synonymous with prescribing opioids.

Clinician perception of the relative importance of pain and its management can also lead to under-treatment. Some health care professionals do not want to routinely accept the patient's self-report of his or her degree of pain as credible. Fear of regulatory scrutiny may also inhibit efforts to control pain.

The inability of the patient to report symptoms accurately, which may occur with cognitively impaired patients, may result in poor communication and a decreased likelihood that the clinician will successfully understand the patient's needs. All of these barriers are associated with a number of myths about pain and its treatment.

THE ROLE OF REFERRAL FOR CONSULTATION IN PAIN MANAGEMENT

The complex nature of pain and its management can be quite challenging. Sometimes even deciding to seek expert consultation in clinical management can be confusing due to a lack of education, fear of regulatory scrutiny, or the absence of consensus or guidelines.[4]

To help clinicians facing these challenges, in 1997 the Federation of State Medical Boards (FSMB) undertook an initiative to develop model guidelines. They encouraged state medical boards and other health care regulatory agencies to adopt policies to encourage adequate and comprehensive pain treatment, including the use of opioids when appropriate for patients with pain. Since the adoption of these model guidelines in April 1998[5], for the use of controlled substances to manage pain, they have been widely distributed to state regulatory agencies and to health care providers. The guidelines have been endorsed by agencies and organizations including the American Pain Society, the American Academy of Pain Medicine, and the Drug Enforcement Administration.

In 2004, the FSMB issued a revised version of the model guidelines[6], renamed as "policy," and commented that despite promulgation of the prior guidelines and other information about the importance of adequately assessing and treating pain, there was increasing concern regarding the abuse, misuse, and diversion of controlled substances. Along with this concern was a body of evidence showing that both acute and chronic pain continued to be under-treated. The under-treatment of pain was recognized as "a serious public health problem that results in a decrease in patients' functional status and quality of life." Identified circumstances that contribute to this problem included:

- Lack of knowledge of:
  - Medical standards with regard to managing pain
  - Current evidence-based research
  - Concrete clinical guidelines for appropriate pain treatment
- Clinical expertise at the level of primary health care providers
- The perception that prescribing adequate amounts of controlled substances may result in unnecessary scrutiny by regulatory authorities
- Misunderstanding of addiction and dependence
- Lack of understanding of regulatory policies and processes

The intention of the FSMB policy and the educational initiatives directed towards expert and non-expert clinicians was clear—to improve the adequacy of pain treatment, while accounting for the issues surrounding appropriate use of modalities and methods in a safe and efficacious manner. Among other often-recommended steps to achieve these goals was the recommendation for the clinician to be *"willing to refer the patient as necessary for additional evaluation and treatment in order to achieve treatment objectives. Special attention should be given to those patients with pain who are at risk for medication misuse, abuse or diversion. The management of pain in patients with a history of substance abuse or with a comorbid psychiatric disorder may require extra care, monitoring, documentation and consultation with or referral to an expert in the management of such patients."*

The rationale for referral to an expert can be multifaceted or focused; sometimes there is a clear reason.

■ *When a comprehensive, multidisciplinary assessment is necessary*

- There may be a persistent pain condition for which there is likely no curative treatment available, and the available methods of management have been exhausted and unsuccessful.

- The referral for an evaluation may be helpful for diagnostic reasons, including interventional diagnostic procedures that go beyond the area of expertise of the primary care clinician.

- Referral may be useful for treatment recommendations, including ongoing management options or symptom control.

- Assistance may be needed to plan further interventions or management.

- An assessment from a specific discipline is considered beneficial (e.g., psychosocial evaluation).

Members of a multidisciplinary pain management team may include:

- Anesthesiologists
- Clergy
- Complementary and Alternative Medicine Specialists
- Neurologists
- Nurses
- Physical Medicine and Rehabilitation Specialists
- Physical or Occupational Therapists
- Psychiatrists
- Psychologists
- Social Workers

Pain clinics may bring all relevant team members "under one roof." Many pain specialists believe that referrals frequently are made past the so-called "golden hour," when their intervention may be of maximal effectiveness, especially in cases of neuropathic and cancer pain.[7] Referral to a pain specialist ideally should occur before significant disability or loss of function occurs; pain behaviors or the emergence of maladaptive coping strategies may serve as cues for referral. Some common reasons for referral include:

■ *An interventional approach is thought to be necessary*

- In certain situations minimally invasive procedures such as epidural steroid injections, nerve root blocks, facet injections, nerve stimulators, and infusion pumps may be indicated for:
  - The purpose of relieving pain directly
  - Diagnostic purposes
  - The intention of improving functional activity and quality of life
  - Intermediary purposes to defer or delay more invasive procedural approaches such as surgery
  - When non-invasive procedures have not yielded the desired goals of treatment

■ *Medical management is thought to require specific expertise beyond the provider's scope of clinical practice*

- The patient may be a management challenge for a number of reasons including:
  - Lack of, or poor response, to treatment regimens that have been tried
  - The patient has been evaluated as an appropriate candidate for opioid therapy, but the opioid risk assessment reveals that the patient is high risk and requires more monitoring than is available
  - The patient's assessment reveals a history of prior or current opioid abuse
  - The patient has specific comorbid conditions needing coordinated care (e.g., depression)

There can also be a benefit to having a fresh, comprehensive review of a patient with chronic pain. This may be a good reason for expert consultation, especially when the treatment plans that have been attempted are not achieving their desired goals.

It is important for the referring clinician to make sure that the patient is adequately informed of the purpose of the referral, *before* the referral, and that appropriate expectations are identified. It is critical that the patient does not have the inaccurate perception that the referral represents disbelief or abandonment by the referring health care provider. On the contrary, it should be emphasized that the consultant involvement will be time-limited., and that the patient's ongoing care will then be provided by his/her primary practitioner again.

There should be discussion and agreement with the patient and the primary care provider about the benefits of maintaining the primary care provider as their care coordinator, and as the source for referrals, rather than engaging in self-referrals or cross-referrals from one specialist to another.[8] Coordinating referrals with the primary care provider as the "medical home" will likely enhance both communication and the quality of care.

REFERENCES

1. Brennan F, Carr DB, Cousins, M. Pain management: a fundamental human right. *Anesth Analg.* 2007;105:(1):205-21.

2. Turk D, Melzack R. *Handbook of Pain Assessment.* 2nd ed. New York: Guilford Press; 2001.

3. Decade of pain control and research. American Pain Society. http://www.ampainsoc.org/decadeofpain

4. Ballantyne JC. *The Massachusetts General Hospital Handbook of Pain Management.* 3rd ed. Philadelphia: Lippincott Williams & Wilkins; October 1, 2005.

5. *Model Guidelines for the Use of Controlled Substances for the Treatment of Pain.* Federation of State Medical Boards of the United States, Inc. April 1998.

6. *Model Policy for the Use of Controlled Substances for the Treatment of Pain* Federation of State Medical Boards of the United States, Inc. Adopted as policy by the House of Delegates of the Federation of State Medical Boards of the United States, Inc., May 2004.

7. Warfield CA, Bajwa ZH. *Principles and Practices of Pain Management.* 2nd ed. New York: McGraw-Hill Companies, Inc; 2004.

8. O'Malley AS, Cunningham PJ. Patient experiences with coordination of care: the benefit of continuity and primary care physician as referral source. *J Gen Intern Med.* 2009 Feb;24(2):170-7.

II.

The Epidemiology of Pain

DEFINITION OF PAIN

The International Association for the Study of Pain (IASP) defines pain as "an unpleasant sensory and emotional experience associated with actual or potential tissue damage."

Pain is a ubiquitous phenomenon. As clinicians know, the same set of circumstances can cause significant pain in one patient and little or none in another. The challenge, then, is not only to identify the type and source of pain a patient is experiencing, but also to assess the severity and impact of the painful condition, in order to ensure optimal treatment. Pain is somewhat of a "black box," in that only the sufferer fully understands the experience. Pain has both subjective and objective components, the proportions of which may be variable, but all of which must be treated. Additionally, consideration must be given to the temporal nature of the pain, as treatment strategies for acute pain may differ dramatically from those for chronic pain.

INCIDENCE AND PREVALENCE OF PAIN

Almost everyone experiences pain at some time in his or her life. In fact, pain is one of the most common reasons for patients to seek medical attention. Of further significance is that more than 50% of the time patients seek treatment from their primary care providers for treatment and diagnosis. On average, 15–20% of Americans experience chronic pain each year, approximately 76 million people. Americans seek advice from a physician on average 3.1 times per year[1], and the majority of these contacts are precipitated by complaints of some type of pain. Pain is associated with wide ranges of injury and disease, and in some situations, is the disease itself. Some conditions may have pain and associated symptoms arising from a discrete cause, such as postoperative pain, or pain associated with pressure related to a tumor. There are also conditions in which pain constitutes the primary problem, such as neuropathic or headache pain. The reality is that when we try to quantify how often it occurs, it can be hard to estimate, as the incidence and prevalence of the associated conditions vary as well.

Furthermore, research shows that the incidence of chronic pain may vary based on a number of different demographic factors such as age, race, and gender[2]. Additionally, many factors have been deemed responsible for disparities in pain assessment, and ultimately treatment in these differing populations as well. (See Chapter VII "Pain Management in Special Patient Populations.") A variety of factors for disparate treatment have been identified, including clinician variability, cultural or gender-based differences, and even clinical setting (e.g., emergency department vs. clinic). In reality, the dynamics of chronic pain among diverse populations, including factors such as employment status, cognition, health care accessibility, health care utilization patterns, and pain coping across various groups are not well understood.[3] This variability can make the quantification of incidence and prevalence difficult.

Surgery is the single largest cause of acute pain in the United States, with approximately 46 million procedures performed each year.[4] The majority of patients in the United States report moderate to severe pain postsurgically, even in the face of current treatments and techniques.

As the American population continues to age, there is an increase in the burden of arthritis pain and chronic joint symptoms in people aged 65 or older.[5] In a 1999 poll, a large proportion of respondents indicated some degree of disability secondary to pain, with two out of three elderly individuals responding that pain kept them from participating in activities. Arthritis is the leading cause of disability, with approximately 39 million medical visits and 500,000 hospitalizations per year.[6] Cancer, the second leading cause of death in America[7], is associated with chronic pain in approximately 67% of patients.[8]

BURDEN OF PAIN ON SOCIETY

Besides the physical, physiologic, and psychosocial effects of pain on individual patients, the financial burden placed on society is tremendous. In 1998, the National Institutes of Health estimated the financial burden of pain to be as much as $100 billion per year in medical expenses, lost wages, and other costs, including lost productivity. This loss of productivity is often largely invisible to employers, because it includes under-performance on the job due to pain, as well as time off the job.[9] Chronic back pain is one of the major causes of absence from work in people under 45 years of age.[10]

The American Productivity Audit, a survey of 28,902 working adults, found the following in relation to pain-related work productivity[11]:

- 52.7% of the work force surveyed reported having headache, back pain, arthritis, or other musculoskeletal pain in the prior 2 weeks.

- 12.7% of the work force lost productive time in a 2-week period due to pain.

- Headache (5.4%) was the most common pain condition prompting lost productive time, followed by back pain (3.2%), arthritis pain (2%), and other musculoskeletal pain (2%).

- Headache produced, on average, 3.5 hours of lost productive time per week.

- Overall, workers lost an average of 4.6 hours per week of productive time due to a pain condition.

- Lost productive time from common painful conditions was estimated by this study to cost $61.2 billion per year.

- 76.6% of lost productive time was explained by reduced work performance, *not absenteeism*.

PATIENT DESCRIPTIONS OF PAIN

Pain is described by patients experiencing it in words that relate to physical sensations, such as "tingling" or "aching," and in emotional words, such as "horrifying" or "terrifying." To illustrate pain, people often use vivid verbal analogies such as "I feel like someone is stabbing me repeatedly and twisting the knife," or "My head is in a vise that is being squeezed tighter and tighter." Behavioral responses, including grimacing, bracing, or rubbing the affected area, result in nonverbal communication about pain. These behaviors, and the accompanying physiologic signs and symptoms of autonomic activation (e.g., tachycardia, tachypnea), are common in acute pain but are uncommon in chronic pain, even when it is severe. Physicians and other health care providers may feel challenged when called on to evaluate and treat painful sensations and the suffering they evoke.

The importance of alleviating the adverse consequences of pain and improving pain treatment globally was recognized by the World Health Organization in 1990. The United States government officially designated 2000–2010 as the "Decade of Pain Control and Research." Pain has now earned the official designation as the "fifth vital sign," and patients are encouraged to understand that they have the right to effective assessment and adequate treatment of pain.[12] Much can be done to improve pain assessment and treatment, as this manual and **www.PainEDU.org** demonstrate.

REFERENCES

1. National Center for Health Statistics. Health, United States, 2006 With Chartbook on Trends in the Health of Americans. Hyattsville, MD: 68-71.

2. Green CA, Anderson KO, Baker TA, et al. The unequal burden of pain: confronting racial and ethnic disparities in pain. *Pain Med.* 2003 Sep;(4):277–94.

3. Ortega RA, Youdelman BA, Havel RC. Ethnic variability in the treatment of pain. *Am J Anesthesiol.* 26(9):429-432.

4. DeFrances CJ, Lucas CA, Buie VC, Golosinskiy A. 2006 National Hospital Discharge Survey. National health statistics reports; no 5. Hyattsville, MD: National Center for Health Statistics. 2008.

5. Centers for Disease Control and Prevention (CDC). Prevalence of disabilities and associated health conditions among adults—United States, 1999. *MMWR Morb Mortal Wkly Rep.* 2001;50:120–125.

6. Centers for Disease Control and Prevention (CDC). Public health and aging: projected prevalence of self-reported arthritis or chronic joint symptoms among persons aged >65 years—United States, 2005–2030. *MMWR Morb Mortal Wkly Rep.* 2003;52:489–491.

7. National Center for Health Statistics. Health, United States, 2009: With Special Feature on Medical Technology. Hyattsville, MD. 2010.

8. Fitzgibbon DR. Cancer pain: management. In: Loeser JD, Butler SH, Chapman CR, Turk DC, eds. *Bonica's Management of Pain.* 3rd ed. Philadelphia: Lippincot, Williams & Wilkins; 2001:659–703.

9. National Institutes of Health. NIH Guide: New Directions in Pain Research I. September 4, 1998.

10. Andersson GB. Epidemiological features of chronic low-back pain. *Lancet.* 1999; Aug 14;(9178):581–5.

11. Stewart WF, Ricci JA, Chee E, et al. Lost productive time and cost due to common pain conditions in the US workforce. *JAMA.* 2003;190:2443–2454.

12. American Pain Foundation Web site. Pain Facts & Figures. http://www.painfoundation.org/newsroom/reporter-resources/pain-facts-figures.html. Accessed April 28, 2010.

III.

Pathophysiology of Pain

MECHANISM OF NORMAL PAIN

In the past, it was thought that a sensory input, such as a pinprick, would cause a pain "signal" to be sent directly to the brain via a single nerve. Although not completely understood today, the science of pain reveals a much more complex process that still is continuing to evolve. New receptors, pathways, and hypotheses are being investigated every day. In addition to identifying new pathways, genetic variations at the receptor level further complicate the treatment process and evaluation of its efficacy. The following is a brief review of basic concepts important to understanding the physiology of pain. For more detailed information on this topic, as well as new developments, visit **www.PainEDU.org.**

THE PAIN PATHWAY

Four steps occur along the pain pathway[1]:

- Transduction
- Transmission
- Modulation
- Perception

**Transduction** is the process by which afferent nerve endings participate in translating noxious stimuli (e.g., a pinprick) into nociceptive impulses. Silent nociceptors, also involved in transduction, are afferent nerves that do not respond to external stimulation unless inflammatory mediators are present. The peripheral nervous system contains primary sensory afferent neurons that have an important role in pain signaling. The axons of these afferents diverge from the cell body in the dorsal root ganglion near the spinal cord and send a short fiber centrally into the cord and a long fiber down the peripheral nerve into the tissues. Their receptors detect mechanical, thermal, proprioceptive, and chemical stimuli. There are three types of primary afferents: A-beta fibers, A-delta fibers, and C-fibers. A-beta fibers are myelinated, large-diameter fibers that respond primarily to light touch and moving stimuli, such as vibration. A-delta fibers (myelinated, small-diameter fibers) and unmyelinated C-fibers respond to noxious (potentially painful) stimuli. Fibers that respond maximally to noxious stimulation are classified as pain fibers, or nociceptors. These are generally A-delta fibers and C-fibers. These nociceptors respond to noxious mechanical, thermal, and chemical stimuli.[2]

Noxious stimulation is first carried by the faster A-delta fibers and then by the slower C-fibers. Local injury can cause nociceptors to become hypersensitive to noxious stimuli, thereby creating a condition called *sensitization*, mediated by algogenic (i.e., pain-generating) substances in the periphery. A sequence of events occurs after local tissue injury, including local vasodilation, edema, and spreading vasodilation (flare), which is known as the *triple response of Lewis*. This is accompanied by *hyperalgesia* (an exaggerated response to painful stimuli) in the injured area (primary hyperalgesia) and hyperalgesia that spreads beyond the injured area (secondary hyperalgesia).[3]

Transmission is the process by which impulses are sent to the dorsal horn of the spinal cord, and then along the sensory tracts to the brain. The primary afferent neurons are active senders and receivers of chemical and electrical signals. Their axons terminate in the dorsal horn of the spinal cord, where they have connections with many spinal neurons. In turn, spinal neurons have inputs from many primary afferents. These spinal neurons project axons to the contralateral thalamus, which in turn projects to the somatosensory pathway, frontal cortex, and other areas. The somatosensory cortex is thought to be involved in the sensory aspects of pain, such as the intensity and quality of pain, whereas the frontal cortex and limbic system are thought to be involved with the emotional responses to it.

The major ascending tract is the spinothalamic tract (STT). Cell bodies of the STT are located primarily in lamina V, but also in laminae I, VII, and VIII. These neurons have axons that cross to the opposite side of the spinal cord and enter its anterolateral quadrant. The STT divides in two different pathways as it approaches the thalamus. The neospinothalamic tract, or lateral STT, is the tract that subserves the sensory/discriminative aspects of pain perception. It synapses on the lateral thalamus and projects to the somatosensory cortex. The medial STT, or paleospinothalamic tract, synapses in the brain stem reticular formation, the medial thalamus, periaqueductal gray matter, and the hypothalamus, and has subsequent projections to the cortex and limbic system. This tract subserves the affective/motivational aspects of pain perception.[3]

Modulation is the process of dampening or amplifying these pain-related neural signals. Modulation takes place primarily in the dorsal horn of the spinal cord, but also elsewhere, with input from ascending and descending pathways. Rich arrays of opioid receptors (mu, kappa, and delta) are present in the dorsal horn. In addition to an ascending tract, the nociceptive system contains descending pathways that send neurons from the frontal cortex and hypothalamus to the midbrain and medulla. These neurons inhibit nociceptive neurons and interneurons in the ascending pathway.[4] Important centers of this descending antinociceptive modulation system are the periventricular and periaqueductal gray matter, the dorsolateral pons, the nucleus raphe magnus, and the rostroventral medulla. Descending pathways project axons to laminae I, II, and V in the spinal cord. In addition to endogenous opioids, the biogenic amines (serotonin and norepinephrine) are neurotransmitters involved in this process. A variety of modalities can activate the descending antinociceptive pathways, including systemic or neuraxial injection of opioids, electric stimulation, stress, suggestion, and pain.[3]

The gate control theory is a popular model of pain modulation proposed by Melzack and Wall in 1965, and was later revised by Melzack and Casey in 1968. These investigators proposed the existence of an endogenous ability to reduce or increase the degree of perceived pain through modulation of incoming impulses at a gate located in the dorsal horn of the spinal cord. The gate acts on signals from the ascending and descending systems and weighs all of the inputs. The integration of these inputs from sensory neurons, the segmental spinal cord level, and the brain determines whether the gate will be opened or closed, either increasing or decreasing the intensity of the ascending pain signal. The importance of psychological variables in the perception of pain, including motivation to escape pain, and the role of thoughts, emotions, and stress reactions in increasing or decreasing painful sensations, is evident in the gate control theory. An example of this is when patients report more pain at night when they are isolated and less distracted from their pain than they might be during the day. The proposed gate can be opened or closed by pharmacologic manipulation, transduction, transmission and modulation, and psychological intervention.

__Perception__ refers to the subjective experience of pain that results from the interaction of transduction, transmission, modulation, and the psychological aspects of the individual.

■ **Table 3.1**
 Normal Pain Pathway at a Glance

Transduction	Transmission	Modulation	Perception
The process by which afferent nerve endings participate in translating noxious stimuli (e.g., a pinprick) into nociceptive impulses	The process by which impulses are sent to the dorsal horn of the spinal cord and then along the sensory tracts to the brain	The process of dampening or amplifying pain-related neural signals, primarily in the dorsal horn of the spinal cord, but also elsewhere, with input from ascending and descending pathways	The subjective experience of feeling pain that results from the interaction of transduction, transmission, modulation, and psychological aspects of the individual

DEFINITION OF ABNORMAL PAIN

Pain associated with the functioning of the unaltered nociceptive system, such as stepping on a thumbtack or touching a hot stove, is referred to as *normal pain* or *nociceptive pain*. Pain that occurs in the context of a nociceptive system that has been altered by tissue damage or other processes may be referred to as *abnormal pain*. There are a number of different ways of classifying abnormal pain, with no universally accepted approach. Following is a classification system that appears to represent emerging consensus.

Inflammatory pain is the sensation that results from injury to a somatic tissue (e.g., skin, muscle, bone), which is invariably followed by an inflammatory reaction. For example, inflammatory pain is felt as the result of an acute injury or infection. The pain produced consequent to tissue inflammation results from a number of different processes. The release in injured tissue of so-called algogenic substances, such as bradykinin and serotonin results in "sensitization" of the peripheral nociceptors, resulting in a lower threshold for firing and an increased frequency of firing compared with their resting state. Sensitization of nociceptive afferents means that these neurons now respond to non-noxious stimuli, such as a light touch or contact with clothing. So-called silent nociceptors may also be recruited; these are nociceptive nerve fibers that normally are silent, but in the setting of inflammation generate "pain" signals. After tissue healing, the pain generally resolves. However, in states of ongoing inflammation, such as rheumatoid arthritis or cancer, pain persists. In cases where inflammation may resolve but leave permanent anatomic alterations, such as the joint damage produced by osteoarthritis, chronic pain may result even though inflammation disappears or becomes inconspicuous.

What mechanisms lead inflammatory pain to become chronic or severe? One proposed mechanism is *central sensitization*, which refers to the process by which, as a consequence of excessive nociceptive nerve signals bombarding the central nervous system from the periphery, long-term changes occur in the central nervous system that result in persistent amplification of pain signals. One experimental paradigm resulting in central sensitization is known as *wind-up*; there are also other pathways to central sensitization. Central sensitization is one proposed mechanism by which in the context of inflammation or nerve injury (see neuropathic pain) normally innocuous stimuli produce pain, such as is seen in many cases of postherpetic neuralgia.[2] The phenomenon of normally innocuous stimuli (such as light touch) producing pain is called *allodynia*.

Central sensitization may also cause an exaggerated response to normally painful stimuli; this is called *hyperalgesia*. *Primary hyperalgesia* occurs at the site of injury and is characterized by a lower pain threshold, spontaneous pain, and increased sensitivity. It usually features thermal and mechanical hypersensitivity.[3] *Secondary hyperalgesia* refers to hyperalgesia occurring outside the area originally injured and is thought usually to be a consequence of central sensitization. The significance of the distinction is that to effectively treat chronic pain, hypersensitivity must be addressed during the clinical assessment of patients. Therapy that targets the mechanisms of hypersensitivity, if present, rather than mechanisms of nociception, must be used to try to alleviate symptoms.[4]

Neuropathic pain is defined as pain due to damaged or dysfunctional nerves. The pathophysiology of neuropathic pain can have both peripheral and central mechanisms. There have been multiple proposed mechanisms for both peripheral and central components to the pathophysiology of neuropathic pain; it is doubtful that a single mechanism can account for all cases. Damaged primary afferents may generate signals at ectopic or abnormal locations and their excitability increases after mechanical stimulation. In addition, nerves that are cut off from input from the periphery, as in the case of amputation, may become hyperactive. Changes in the dorsal horn after nerve injury include reorganization, modulation in sensory input, enlargement of the second-order neuron's receptive field, alteration in opioid receptivity, abnormal ingrowth of sympathetic nerve terminals, and abnormal temporal summation.[5] Thus, central nervous system changes, as well as peripheral nerve changes, may generate neuropathic pain.

Woolf and Mannion categorize peripheral neuropathic pain as either spontaneous (*stimulus-independent*) or hypersensitive (*stimulus-evoked*) because of increased sensitivity after damage to sensory neurons.[6]

Dysfunctional pain refers to a pain syndrome in which patients experience pain and abnormal sensitivity not associated with noxious stimulus, tissue damage, inflammation, or identifiable lesion to the nervous system. The conditions encompassed by dysfunctional pain may include fibromyalgia, tension-type headaches, migraines, and even irritable bowel syndrome. Individuals with these syndromes share a number of common characteristics, including hyper-vigilance to sensory stimuli, exaggerated experience of a diverse array of sensory stimuli (e.g., pain, but also sound, light, etc.), high prevalence of associated conditions (e.g., the high prevalence of irritable bowel syndrome in patients with fibromyalgia), and, in some cases, abnormal biomarkers (e.g., opioid peptides in spinal fluid).

There are many other ways of describing pain and terms that support them. An important term is *referred pain*, the perception of pain in a body part in which it did not originate (e.g., feeling pain from the diaphragm near the shoulder).The mechanism of referred pain is thought to be convergence of primary afferents from different locations (e.g., shoulder and diaphragm) onto the same spinal cord neurons. Because spinal neurons subserve both deep structures and skin, mislocation of sensations is possible.

Classification of pain into different types and mechanisms is more than just academic interest. Data continue to emerge indicating that different types of pain respond to different types of treatment, so that accurate classification of the type of pain can support accurate selection of treatment.

Additionally, when considering formulating a treatment plan that includes opioid analgesics, it is important to consider that new research shows that variations in patient response may be genetically-based at the receptor level. Most of the opioids used in clinical practice exert their effects through mu opioid receptors. Their potency, effectiveness, and adverse effects can vary unpredictably among patients. Researchers feel that these variations "strongly argue against a single receptor mediating their actions".[7] A single mu opioid receptor gene has been identified, but current thinking is that there are numerous mu opioid receptor subtypes that are in part responsible for this variation in response.

There is a need to individualize therapy for each and every patient in order to maximize the safety and efficacy of pain treatment. Consideration of variation in pain conditions themselves, metabolic differences with regard to cytochrome P-450, and genetic receptor polymorphism, further reinforces that need.

REFERENCES

1. Katz WA. *Pain Management in Rheumatologic Disorders: A Guide for Clinicians*. N.p.: Drugsmartz; 2000.

2. Fields HL, Basbaum AI. Central nervous system mechanisms of pain modulation. In: Wall PD, Melzack R, eds. *Textbook of Pain*. London: Churchill; 2000:309–330.

3. Raj PP. Pain mechanisms. In: Raj PP, ed. *Pain Medicine: A Comprehensive Review*. 1st ed. Missouri: Mosby-Year Book; 1996:12–23.

4. Mannion RJ, Woolf CJ. Pain mechanisms and management: a central perspective. *Clin J Pain*. 2000;16(Suppl 3):S144–S156.

5. Galer BS, Dworkin RH. *A Clinical Guide to Neuropathic Pain*. New York: McGraw Hill, Healthcare Information Programs; 2000.

6. Woolf CJ, Mannion RJ. Neuropathic pain: etiology, symptoms, mechanisms, and management. *Lancet*. 1999;353:1959–1964.

7. Pasternak GW. Molecular insights into mu opioid pharmacology: From the clinic to the bench. *Clin J Pain*. 2010 Jan;26 Suppl 10:S3-9.

IV.

Pain Assessment

DEFINITIONS

Regardless of whether pain is thought to be nociceptive, neuropathic, or idiopathic, it is also usually broadly categorized as either *acute* or *chronic*. Additionally, pain is also categorized based on other characteristics, such as its intensity, location, quality, and factors that alleviate or worsen it.

Some simple distinguishing characteristics of acute and chronic pain include the following:

- **Acute pain**
  - Generally sudden onset, certainly recent onset
  - *Usually* has an obvious identifiable cause
    - Injury
    - Disease
    - Iatrogenic (e.g., surgery)
  - Short duration (less than 1 month)
  - Intensity generally variable and indicative of severity of underlying condition or situation
  - Characteristic behavior, such as rubbing, moaning, crying

- **Chronic pain**
  - Persistent (generally 3 months duration or longer), often undetermined onset

- *Usually* the result of some chronic disease, condition, or situation
- May have no obvious cause
- Prolonged functional impairment
  - Physical
  - Psychological
- May or may not be associated with characteristic behavior, such as insomnia, anorexia, irritability, and depression
- Often more difficult to manage than acute pain

Basic Terminology

Acute pain is the result of an injury or illness that is time-limited and of recent onset. Low back pain after an injury, acute headache, and postoperative pain are examples of acute pain. Acute pain is generally thought to have the biologic function of alerting the individual to harm and preparing for the "fight-or-flight" response to danger. It is an important part of the vital, protective sentry system that permits us to live in an environment filled with potential dangers. Diagnosing and treating the underlying cause of pain, in addition to treating the symptomatic pain, are the critical elements of pain management. *Subacute pain* is pain that usually lasts up to 3 months.

Baseline pain is generally constant in nature and lasts at least half of the day.

Breakthrough pain increases over baseline pain to a significantly higher degree of intensity. Incident pain is a type of breakthrough pain that increases with activity or movement.

Central pain is initiated or caused by a primary lesion or dysfunction in the central nervous system.

Chronic pain persists and does not resolve spontaneously. Chronic pain has usually been defined *arbitrarily* as pain that persists for 3–6 months or longer, or beyond the period of expected healing. Ongoing or progressive tissue damage may be present in some types of chronic pain, including progressive neuropathic pain and rheumatologic conditions. In other cases, chronic pain may be present when tissue damage is stable or undetectable.

Neuralgia is pain along the distribution of a nerve or nerves.

Neurogenic pain is initiated or caused by a primary lesion, dysfunction, or transitory irritation in the peripheral or central nervous system.

Neuropathic pain is initiated or caused by a primary lesion or dysfunction in the nervous system. *Peripheral neuropathic pain* occurs when the lesion or dysfunction affects the peripheral nervous system. *Central neuropathic pain* may be also referred to as *central pain* when the lesion or dysfunction affects the central nervous system.

Pain Categorized by Source and Related Nociceptor

Cutaneous pain is caused by injury to skin or superficial tissues. Cutaneous nociceptors terminate just below the skin and have a high concentration of nerve endings, producing well-localized pain.

Somatic pain originates from somatic nociceptors, located in structures such as ligaments, bones, and blood vessels. The low concentration of nerve endings results in a dull, poorly localized pain sensation that is usually of longer duration than cutaneous pain.

Visceral pain originates from organ-level nociceptors located within the organs themselves or visceral cavities. Visceral nociceptors exist in even lower concentrations than somatic or cutaneous nociceptors, resulting in even more elusive qualities with respect to localization. The quality of visceral pain is typically more of a diffuse aching pain of longer duration.

Assessment

To begin an assessment, all patients should be asked about the presence of current pain or of pain over the past several months. Clinicians often ask, *"How can I know how much pain my patient is feeling?"* Unfortunately, there are no objective tests that can indicate the precise quality and intensity of pain and tease out the patient's affective and behavioral reactions to it. Because of the multiple dimensions of pain, it is considered to be a *purely subjective experience*.

There are, however, standardized measures and clinical questions that can be used to assess pain and associated symptoms, such as sleep disturbance and functional status. These measures rely primarily on the patient's self-report, which, despite limitations, remains the single most reliable indicator of the existence and intensity of pain. Techniques to assess pain when self-report is unavailable or unreliable are introduced in Chapter VII. In this section, several commonly used measures of pain intensity are reviewed, as are clinical interview questions that form part of the pain assessment. Important points of assessment in the physical examination and thorough diagnostic testing also are included.

Careful and accurate assessment of pain is critical for successful diagnosis and treatment. Some important first steps include identifying key points with respect to the patient's pain:

- The **description** of painful symptoms (e.g., burning, throbbing)

- The **location** of the pain

- The **temporal nature** of the pain
  - Acute versus chronic
  - Time of occurrence and duration

- The **severity** of the pain
  - Impact on activities of daily living
  - Psychological impact
  - Social impact

- **Exacerbating** (e.g., bending) and/or **alleviating** (e.g., ice) **factors**

- **Steps taken** before presenting for management
  - Reduction in activity
  - Medication use before visit

It is also important to consider that *pain assessment is not a one-time phenomenon.* According to the Joint Commission standards for 2001[1] pain is considered to be *the fifth vital sign* and should be assessed initially and reassessed on a scheduled and regular basis. The National Comprehensive Cancer Network set these guidelines for severe cancer pain in 2010[2]:

■ Patients receiving intravenous short-acting opioids should be assessed every 15 minutes for rapid titration.

■ Patients receiving administered short-acting opioids should be assessed every 60 minutes.

■ Patients receiving long-acting opioids should be reassessed at least every dosing cycle.

Patients should be informed of the need for regular pain assessment, and told that a score above a predetermined level will be therapeutically addressed.

PATIENT HISTORY

Much of the information the clinician gleans about the patient's pain complaint is gained in a thorough history and physical examination. The following sample questions should be included as part of a thorough clinical history evaluation:

■ **What is the location, quality, and frequency of pain?**

  ■ In addition to pointing to the **location of the pain** and a verbal description, the patient can draw the location of pain on a body diagram.

  ■ **Primary and secondary sites** should be elicited because patients often experience more than one location of pain. In addition, the patient can be asked to assign the percentage of pain in each area relative to the overall pain experienced.

  ■ Diagnostic information can be obtained by asking about the **quality of pain**. For example, neuropathic pain is often described as "tingling, burning, or shooting," whereas visceral pain is often described as "dull, aching, or squeezing."

  ■ The **frequency of pain** can be constant, intermittent, or cyclic, with exacerbations that occur over and above a consistent level of pain.

- The **presence and timing of exacerbations** may indicate the need for increased analgesic medication or nonpharmacologic interventions.

■ **What are the variations and patterns of pain? What factors alleviate or worsen pain?**

- **Patterns of pain** can be helpful in diagnosis and treatment. For example, patients with consistent patterns of morning pain can have their medication regimen adjusted to help them accomplish morning routines. The **temporal pattern of pain**—that is, whether it is constant or intermittent, sudden, or gradual—is one of the most important elements in the medical history that leads to diagnosis.

- **Provocative factors**, such as activities like bending forward or backward, may also be helpful in determining the differential diagnosis. **Relief maneuvers**, such as bed rest, or activity modification are important as well.

■ **When was the onset of pain? What is the history of pain management interventions? How did each of these interventions work?**

- The **onset** of pain, both in terms of the **duration** of pain and the manner in which the pain occurred (acute, accident, insidious), has implications for treatment and may hold meaning for the patient. For example, an insidious onset of pain with an unexplained etiology may have different implications in terms of seeking treatment and coping with pain.

- Patients should also be asked about **prior use of pharmacologic, nonpharmacologic, and procedural interventions** for pain. The patient may have used alternative or complementary medical approaches, such as herbal preparations, acupuncture, or magnets. The relief experienced from each of these interventions can be measured by using a visual analogue scale (VAS) or by asking the patient to assign a percentage value of relief (e.g., 50% pain relief from the use of nonsteroidal anti-inflammatory drugs) for each treatment.

■ **What are the physical limitations resulting from the pain?**

■ Patients are generally quick to describe their **functional limitations** due to pain. Walking, performing domestic chores, or continuing to work in their occupation may all be affected. Individuals in acute pain may be unable to turn over, cough, or breathe deeply, secondary to their pain. Special attention should be paid to the ways patients compensate for their inability to perform physical tasks, such as walking. Be aware that compensation with another limb (e.g., performing all duties with one hand), can lead to overuse syndromes and/ or more serious problems in previously unaffected areas.

■ **What are the expectations of treatment?**

■ Patients may have high or unrealistic expectations for treatment. Although the probability that these expectations can be met in an acute setting is high, the probability may decrease for chronic pain conditions.

■ The urgency of treatment and the expectations for it may be based on inaccurate assumptions or beliefs, such as that pain signifies ongoing damage or the return of a cancerous tumor. **Patient education** about the underlying cause of the pain and the effectiveness of medications, interventional procedures, and nonpharmacologic treatments should be delivered carefully and honestly in lay language. **Setting appropriate expectations** of treatment can itself be of therapeutic benefit.

PHYSICAL EXAMINATION FOR PAIN

The physical examination for patients with pain should include a general physical, as well as neurologic, musculoskeletal, and mental assessments, and it is likely to be a more complex process than that of other medical patients.[2] In addition, the examination should involve an assessment of the patient's functional abilities. A careful examination of the site of the patient's pain, including anatomic sites of commonly referred pain, should also be performed. The general appearance of the patient, including attributes of the skin, posture, and demeanor, are important aspects of the general physical examination.

Musculoskeletal Examination

The musculoskeletal examination includes an overall examination and focused palpation, or manipulation, at the site of pain. The examination needs to be tailored to the pain complaint. Muscle systems in the neck, upper extremities, trunk, and lower extremities, should be tested.[3] Deep or superficial muscle tenderness should be noted. The quality of the patient's response to palpation may be considered in the assessment. Vocalizations or a display of pain behavior may be part of the patient's cultural and/or ethnic background and can be of importance when a more stoic individual displays pain behavior in response to palpation.[3] Range of motion, including flexion, extension, side bending, rotating, and straight-leg raises, should be performed when relevant to ascertain whether pain is experienced on movement, and to note the presence of functional restrictions. The degree to which these actions are performed, and whether pain is incurred during each of these exercises, should be recorded.

Neurologic Examination

A tailored neurologic examination is a key component of the physical examination for pain. The neurologic screening examination should include standard elements, with testing of the cranial nerves II–XII. Motor and sensory functioning in the limbs and an evaluation of rectal and urinary sphincter function have been recommended. Sensory deficits are tested by sensitivity to light touch, pinprick, and mechanical and thermal stimuli. Light touch, pressure, or the application of hot and cold stimuli can cause *allodynia*—that is, the presence of pain from a stimulus that is not normally painful. *Hyperalgesia*, or extreme pain from stimuli that normally do cause pain, can be tested by single and multiple pinpricks, and is evidence of pathology. A motor examination should test for motor weakness, ataxia, apraxia, and decreased endurance.[4] Reflexes should be normal and symmetric. In addition, pathologic reflexive signs, such as those of Babinski, Oppenheim, Gordon, Chaddock, Schaeferand, and Hoffman, should be tested when relevant.

DIAGNOSTIC TESTING

Diagnostic testing can be useful for some pain conditions and may not be useful in other types of pain conditions. Therefore, familiarity with general principles of diagnostic testing is important when assessing patients with pain.

Imaging Studies

Imaging studies show anatomy, not pain. Thus, there may be false-positives where "abnormalities" are revealed that are unrelated to the patient's pain, or false-negatives where the anatomy is "normal," yet pain continues. Computed tomography myelogram, magnetic resonance imaging, ultrasound, and radionuclide examinations are used in patients with pain to confirm or rule out a diagnosis, based on the patient's report and the physician's assessment. In the presence of certain signs and symptoms, such as an extremely severe headache or a history of malignancy, imaging can be critical to diagnosis and treatment. Imaging is appropriate for potentially serious spinal conditions, including spinal tumor, fracture, and cauda equina syndrome. Imaging studies are necessary for chronic pain conditions (e.g., unremitting cervical or back pain) for which surgery is being considered. However, imaging plays a limited role in some chronic pain conditions. Because suspected pathologic conditions, such as herniated or bulging disks and nerve root scarring, are frequently found in asymptomatic individuals, the need for imaging studies, and interpretation of results, must be carefully considered, lest they result in inappropriate interventions for irrelevant pathology, or in distraction from the real cause of the pain.

Neurophysiology Studies

Electromyography and nerve conduction studies are electro-diagnostic procedures that evaluate action potentials and conduction along peripheral sensory and motor nerves. They are used to suggest the presence or absence of nerve entrapment, radiculopathy, trauma, and systemic neurologic disease.[5] These tests can provide useful information in the evaluation of the cause and extent of peripheral nervous system disease, but they are often unnecessary in the diagnosis of neuropathic pain conditions. Because they measure the functioning of large nerve fibers, they are not useful in diagnosing many neuropathic conditions that result from small-fiber damage or dysfunction.[4] Quantitative sensory testing measures the function of large and small nerve fibers in addition to pain thresholds. The technique is currently used for researching the mechanisms of neuropathic pain and is generally not needed for diagnosis and treatment. Analogous to the case of imaging, electromyography/nerve conduction studies show nerve damage, not pain; thus, electromyography/nerve conduction studies may be abnormal but unrelated to the pain, or normal in the presence of pain.

MEASURING PAIN INTENSITY

Knowledge of the patient's current pain intensity is important, as are pain intensity levels over time. Questions about pain intensity generally include a timeline (from a week to a month), a parameter (average, least, most), and a rating of pain. Asking about the least and most pain that the patient has experienced over some period of time can establish whether a range of pain exists.

Unidimensional Scales

Two common assessment instruments that can be used to measure pain intensity are the visual analogue scale and the numerical rating scale.

Visual Analogue Scale

The VAS is a 10-cm line with anchors at both ends. Common anchors are "no pain" and "worst pain." Patients are asked to draw a vertical line through the horizontal line to indicate their pain intensity. The line is measured in millimeters, yielding a number between 0 and 100. Research has shown the sensitivity, validity, and reliability of the VAS scale.[6] An example (not to scale) is shown below:

What is the intensity of your pain right now?

|————————————————————————————————————|
0   100
No pain   Worst pain

Numerical Rating Scale

The numerical rating scale (NRS), sometimes referred to as a verbal rating scale (VRS), is an 11-point scale on which patients rate the intensity of their pain by choosing a number from 0, (no pain), to 10 (pain as bad as it could be). This rating scale is commonly used and easy to understand. The scale can be administered visually or verbally, including over the telephone, which can be useful during the dosage titration process.

What is the intensity of your pain right now?

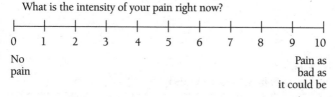

|——+——+——+——+——+——+——+——+——+——|
0   1   2   3   4   5   6   7   8   9   10
No   Pain as
pain   bad as
                                                     it could be

Some investigators prefer the VAS because of certain theoretical psychometric advantages. Others prefer the NRS because fewer patients fail to understand its usage, it is easier to score, and for practical purposes, the psychometric properties work well. A recent survey of 85 chronic pain patients was performed using both the VAS and verbal rating scale.[7] The results of this one survey concluded that comparatively, "the [verbal rating scale] is a simple instrument that can save time and compares favorably to the VAS." Some suggestions for increasing the ease with which patients use the numerical rating scale have been proposed[8] and are also useful in explaining the VAS. The pain scale (e.g., the NRS, VAS) should be explained each time it is administered, and patients should be taught how to use the scale. Patients can be taught that a "10" rating means the worst possible pain. This orientation can reduce the exclusive use of the higher end of the scale and increase the practical application of the measurement. Additional aids can be used to ensure that the patients with hearing or visual difficulties can use the measure with relatively little difficulty. In addition, a quiet place should be provided for the completion of this instrument, and the patient should be allowed to ask questions.[8]

Categorical Scales

Below are two examples of verbal categorical pain scales that provide a simple means for patients to rate their pain intensity using verbal or visual descriptions of their pain.

Simple Descriptive Pain Intensity Scale

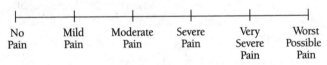

| No Pain | Mild Pain | Moderate Pain | Severe Pain | Very Severe Pain | Worst Possible Pain |

■ **Figure 1**
Faces Pain Scale – REVISED (FPS-R)

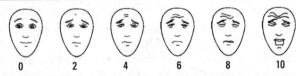

0   2   4   6   8   10

"These faces show how much something can hurt. This face *[point to left-most face]* shows no pain. The faces show more and more pain *[point to each from left to right]* up to this one *[point to right-most face]* – it shows very much pain. Point to the face that shows how much you hurt *[right now]*."

Hicks CL, von Baeyer CL, Spafford P, van Korlaar I, Goodenough B. Faces Pain Scale-Revised: Toward a Common Metric in Pediatric Pain Measurement. PAIN 2001; 93:173-183. With the instructions and translations as found on the web site: www.painsourcebook.ca. This figure has been reproduced with permission of the International Association for the Study of Pain® (IASP®). The figure may not be reproduced for any other purpose without permission.

These unidimensional and categorical pain rating scales remain useful screening tests that should be supplemented frequently by a more detailed assessment.

Multidimensional Tools

Multidimensional pain assessment tools provide information about the pain's characteristics and impact on daily life. The following are three examples of commonly used multidimensional tools for pain assessment in use today.

Initial Pain Assessment Tool

The Initial Pain Assessment Tool was developed for the initial patient pain evaluation. This tool includes a diagram of different body locations so that the patient can mark the areas that correspond to the location of his or her pain. In addition, the following topics are covered in the evaluation:

- Intensity of pain
- Quality of pain (in the patient's own words)
- Onset
- Duration
- Variations
- Presence of rhythmic nature
- Manner of expression of pain
- What, if anything, relieves the pain
- What causes or increases the pain
- What impact the pain has on the patient
  - Accompanying symptoms
  - Sleep
  - Appetite
  - Physical activity
  - Interpersonal relationships
  - Emotional state
  - Ability to concentrate

- Any other pertinent points
- Care plan

Brief Pain Inventory

The Brief Pain Inventory is easy to use and helps to quantify pain intensity and interference with a patient's life. Patients rate their pain severity at its worst, least, and average in the last week and at the time of assessment ("right now").

Brief pain inventory items include the following:

- A diagram of a front and back view of a human figure to identify the location of pain

- A rating of the amount of relief the patient feels that the current pain treatments (if any) provide

- A rating of the duration of the patient's pain relief after taking prescribed pain medications

- An assessment of the patient's attribution of pain to the disease, the treatment of the disease, or conditions unrelated to the disease

Patients also rate their level of pain interference in the following seven contexts from 0 ("does not interfere") to 10 ("completely interferes"):

- Work
- Activity
- Mood
- Enjoyment
- Sleep
- Walking
- Relationships

McGill Pain Questionnaire

The McGill Pain Questionnaire is one of the most extensively used pain scales. The questionnaire consists primarily of three major classes of word descriptors—sensory, affective, and evaluative—that are used by patients to specify their subjective pain experience. It also contains an intensity scale and other items to determine the properties of the pain experience.

The questionnaire was designed to provide quantitative measures of clinical pain that can be treated statistically. The three major measures are the following:

1. The pain rating index, based on two types of numerical values that can be assigned to each word descriptor

2. The number of words chosen

3. The present pain intensity based on a 1–5 intensity scale

Memorial Pain Assessment Card

The Memorial Pain Assessment Card[9] was developed as a rapid multidimensional tool in cancer patients that uses three separate VASs to assess pain, pain relief, and mood. This tool includes a set of adjectives for pain intensity as well. The major advantage of this tool is that it takes very little time to administer; the results also correlate with other, more time-consuming evaluators of pain and mood. The convenience of this card is that it can be carried easily in the clinician's pocket and conveniently presented to the patient, one scale at a time.

■ **Figure 2**
Memorial Pain Assessment Card

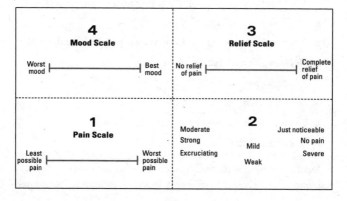

PSYCHOSOCIAL EVALUATION

Pain affects the patient in many ways psychologically and socially. An overall gestalt of the most salient emotional aspects of pain can be elicited by posing a general question about the patient's well-being, such as, "How is the pain affecting your life?" or "How are you coping with your pain and its effect on your life?" Following are some of the more common areas where patients' concerns may lie.

Emotional Reactions

A variety of emotional reactions can be elicited by persistent pain. Identifying negative emotional content and assessing patients' ability to cope with these emotions are critical to improving their functioning. Asking patients, "What's your mood generally like?" may elicit some of the following:

- Anger: often expressed as frustration, irritability, disgust
- Grief: sadness, blue, loss, "I'm not me"
- Depression: anhedonia (lack of pleasure), anergia (lack of energy), loss of interest
- Anxiety: nervous, restless, push to be "fixed"

Patients may experience negative emotions about the following:

- Their circumstances (an injury or accident)
- Their diagnosis (cancer, chronic pain)
- The inability to perform tasks previously performed with ease
- Not being able to "handle" pain
- Treatment providers
- Insurance coverage
- The inability to return to previous job
- A terminal illness

Suicidal ideation is relatively common in patients with chronic pain conditions and should be assessed in every patient and addressed immediately. The risk of death by suicide is estimated to be at least double for patients with chronic pain, compared with controls.[10]

Warning Signs for Referral to a Mental Health Professional

- Suicidal ideation with or without intent or plan
- Anergia
- Persistent anhedonia
- Loss of appetite
- Sleep disturbance
- Anxiety or panic
- Prolonged difficulty accepting the condition
- Angry outbursts toward self or others

Cognitions, Coping, and Beliefs about Pain

Cognitions, or thoughts the patient has, exert powerful effects on emotional reactions, behavioral responses, and interpretations of pain. Beliefs are a foundation for cognitions. For example, the belief that the etiology of pain can be "fixed" or "cured" affects expectations of and satisfaction with treatment. Some maladaptive beliefs and cognitions according to research include the following:

- *Catastrophizing: a cognitive and emotional process that involves magnification of pain-related stimuli, feelings of helplessness, and a negative orientation to pain and life circumstances.*[11] Examples of catastrophic statements include "I can't handle this pain," "There is nothing I can do about my pain," and "My pain is uncontrollable." The effect of catastrophizing should not be underestimated. Catastrophizing is associated with depression, decreases in physical functioning, increased pain,[12] risk of death by suicide,[10] and interpersonal distress.[13] Recent studies suggest that catastrophizing may be related to cortical responses to pain[14] and, potentially, inflammatory disease activity.[11] Catastrophizing predicts poor outcomes for patients with chronic pain and should be treated with cognitive-behavioral therapy.

■ *Belief that persistent pain signals ongoing tissue damage.* This belief results in fear of movement, physical activity, and the future. It may be necessary to educate the patient that pain does not equal harm and that appropriate physical activity is important.

■ *Belief that if a cause of pain can be found, a treatment will fix it.* Patients are generally socialized to believe that medicine has a cure for their problems. Many believe that once a cause of the pain can be found, a treatment that results in a cure is likely (e.g., removing a problematic disk always resolves pain). For many, accepting that chronic pain can be managed but not necessarily cured is a gradual process. Encouragement to continue to be engaged in life as pain is being managed and not wait for a "cure" is often necessary.

■ *Belief that pain is a signal to stop activities and movement.* Some patients believe that pain means that they should rest and be inactive. Social activities may be curtailed or stopped because they feel pain. Although patients may not be able to perform the same physical activities as before, they should be encouraged to do as much as possible because physical inactivity increases pain.[15]

Constructive coping styles, such as using coping self-statements and increasing behavioral activities, have been shown to be more effective ways to manage chronic pain[16] than passive coping strategies (e.g., resting).

The patient should be asked how he or she generally copes with pain, both cognitively (e.g., "What do you tell yourself when you are having a pain flare-up?") and behaviorally (e.g., "What do you do when you are having a pain flare-up?"). Increases in drug, tobacco, and alcohol use, or taking more medication than is prescribed, can be other maladaptive ways of coping with pain, which can lead to an exacerbation of the difficulties in the patient's life.

Behavioral Reactions

Verbal and nonverbal expressions of pain include a range of behaviors, such as the following:

- Grimacing
- Rubbing the affected body part
- Guarding or restricting movement
- Sighing
- Groaning, wailing
- Taking medications
- Resting

These behaviors are *overt* and are called pain behaviors. They can be used to do the following:

- Communicate distress
- Cope with pain
- Elicit solicitous behavior from others
- Express pain in a culturally learned or valued manner
- Express pain when verbal skills are absent or impaired

The frequency with which pain behaviors are displayed, as well as an evaluation of the environmental responses received, may be helpful in assessing whether these expressions are adaptive or maladaptive in a particular circumstance. The expression of pain behaviors may be critical when an individual is unable to express pain verbally (e.g., children, cognitively impaired individuals).

Some behaviors (e.g., resting, taking medication) are problematic when used exclusively as a pain-coping strategy. Sleep disturbance, including insomnia and middle-of-the-night awakening, initially related to painful exacerbations, can become conditioned behavioral responses over time.

Family Functioning and Responses to Pain

The family system is affected when one person becomes unable to function in the expected manner. The responses of family members have been categorized in three ways[17]:

1. Solicitous (e.g., providing assistance or special attention to the patient)

2. Punishing (e.g., becoming angry when pain is expressed)

3. Distracting (e.g., encouraging the patient to distract from the pain)

Research has shown that overly solicitous behaviors or punitive responses from family members or friends are generally not helpful. Research with patients with cancer pain and their families reveals that misconceptions about cancer and pain control on the part of the family have an adverse effect on patient care and outcome.[18]

Those with pain may not be able to fulfill role behavior they perceive as important to their definition of themselves as fathers, mothers, or members of a family or friendship network. For example, a father may not be able to participate in athletic activities with his children and may define this ability as an important part of his role as a father. Families may need assistance changing roles and learning to interact with a person with chronic pain on a long-term basis.

Social and Occupational Functioning

The nature and extent of some chronic pain conditions impact the ability to work and interact in social settings. The stress that accompanies the loss of work involves the loss of a sense of purpose, as well as loss of financial compensation.

Work-related injuries are particularly difficult for workers who believed they were valued employees who became relegated to a "disabled" status after their injury. The process of workers' compensation is complex and sometimes adversarial. Patients might experience the following:

- Be required to participate in independent medical examinations by nontreating physicians to review the appropriateness of treatment

- Be followed by private investigators who routinely investigate claims for fraud

- Be disregarded by coworkers because the pain cannot be seen and the patient "looks good"

- Be sent back to work prematurely

- Be asked to interview for other positions

- Be treated differently by physicians because of their litigation status
- Be denied treatment the treating physician has recommended
- Be financially stressed because of the loss of full-time salary or wages

Patients sometimes feel disbelieved and may feel accused of faking an injury or illness for the purpose of personal gain (e.g., obtaining time off) or malingering. Of course, this process is made difficult for clinicians and patients because a few patients are malingerers. Malingering involves the intentional production of false or grossly exaggerated physical or psychological symptoms for the purpose of tangible external incentives, such as obtaining financial compensation, evading criminal prosecution, avoiding work or military duty, and obtaining drugs.[19]

The presence of workers' compensation or litigation status does not mean the patient does not want to improve and return to work or is demonstrating malingering, although these factors may complicate recovery. Evaluating the obstacles to recovery or rehabilitation (e.g., the patient does not want to return to a former job or employer) and addressing these obstacles during treatment (e.g., with vocational counseling) are important components of treating patients with chronic pain.

Psychiatric Disorders and Pain

Painful conditions, like all medical conditions, affect patients with psychiatric disorders. Selected psychiatric disorders are found in greater prevalence in medical settings and in persons with chronic illnesses. Persons with chronic pain are most often diagnosed with depression, anxiety, and substance-use disorders.[20] Consider the following statistics for individuals meeting criteria for major depressive disorder:

- 2% of people in the community[21]
- 5–9% in ambulatory care[21]
- 15–20% of medical inpatients[21]
- 0–58% of persons with cancer[22]
- 43% with nondisabling pain and depression in primary care[23]
- 66% with disabling pain and depression in primary care[23]

A Word about Somatization Disorder

Some psychiatric disorders have as a primary characteristic the existence of abnormal illness behavior and are therefore more likely to present in medical settings. For example, somatization disorder is characterized by the following:

- A pattern of multiple physical complaints
- Significant social and occupational impairment
- Symptoms that occur before age 30
- Symptoms that last for a period of years
- Pervasive complaints unaccounted for by a general medical condition, including the following:
  - Four different pain symptoms
  - Two gastrointestinal symptoms
  - One sexual symptom and
  - One pseudoneurologic symptom[19]

Although the presence of unexplained somatic symptoms is common, somatization disorder is rare.[21]

The diagnosis of undifferentiated somatoform disorder is less restrictive than somatization disorder, requiring one or more physical complaints that cannot be explained by a general medical condition and that cause significant social or occupational distress. Care should be taken before labeling patients with somatoform disorder or as "somatizers" because of current limitations of diagnostic testing and disease criteria.[21]

Pilowsky[24] suggests that a hallmark of abnormal illness behavior is extreme difficulty accepting advice from a physician if it doesn't fit the patient's appraisal of his or her health status. Avoidance of dualism in pain (i.e., the pain is either in the body or the mind) is key in assessing and treating individuals with pain conditions, and is especially pertinent when treating individuals with psychiatric illnesses.

■ **Table 4.1**

**Summary: General Clinical Questions
to Ask to Assess Psychosocial Aspects of Pain**

Psychosocial Aspects of Pain	Clinical Questions to Ask
Global question	How is the pain affecting your life?
Emotional reactions	What's your mood generally like?
Suicidal thoughts	Do you ever feel like giving up? Do you have suicidal thoughts?
Cognitions, coping, beliefs about pain	How do you cope with the pain?
Behavioral reactions	What do you do when you have a flare up of pain?
Family functioning	How do your family members/supportive others respond when you have pain?
Social and occupational functioning	How are work and social activities going?

REFERENCES

1. Hadjistavropoulos HD, Clark J. Using outcome evaluations to assess interdisciplinary acute and chronic pain programs. *Jt Comm J Qual Improv.* 2001 Jul;27(7):335-48.

2. 2010 NCCN Pain Guidelines http://www.nccn.org/index.asp. Accessed July 21, 2010.

3. Irving GA, Squire PL. Medical evaluation of the chronic pain patient. In: Fishman SM, Ballantyne JC, Rathmell JP, eds. *Bonica's Management of Pain.* 4th ed. Philadelphia: Lippincott Williams & Wilkins; 2009:209-224.

4. Galer BS, Dworkin RH. *A Clinical Guide to Neuropathic Pain.* New York: McGraw Hill Healthcare Information Programs; 2000.

5. Chang DG, Date ES. Electrodiagnostic evaluation of acute and chronic pain syndromes. In: Fishman SM, Ballantyne JC, Rathmell JP, eds. *Bonica's Management of Pain*. 4th ed. Philadelphia: Lippincott Williams & Wilkins, 2009:225-234.

6. Jensen MP, Karoly P. Self-report scales and procedures for assessing pain in adults. In: Turk DC, Melzack R, eds. *Handbook of Pain Assessment*. 2nd ed. New York: Guilford Press, 2001:15-34.

7. Cork RC, Isaac I, Elsharydah A, Saleemi S, Zavisca F, Alexander L. A comparison of the verbal rating scale and the visual analog scale for pain assessment. *Internet J Anesthesiol*. 2004;8(1).

8. Clark ME, Gironda RJ, Young RW. Development and validation of the Pain Outcomes Questionnaire-VA. *J Rehabil Res Dev*. 2003 Sep-Oct;40(5):381-95.

9. Fishman B, Pasternak S, Wallenstein SL, et al. The Memorial Pain Assessment Card. A valid instrument for the evaluation of cancer pain. *Cancer*. 1987 Sep 1;60(5):1151-8.

10. Tang NK, Crane C. Suicidality in chronic pain: a review of the prevalence, risk factors and psychological links. *Psychol Med*. 2006;36:575–586.

11. Edwards RR, Bingham CO 3rd, Bathon J, Haythornthwaite JA. Catastrophizing and pain in arthritis, fibromyalgia, and other rheumatic diseases. *Arthritis Rheum*. 2006;55:325–332.

12. Bishop SR, Warr D. Coping, catastrophizing and chronic pain in breast cancer. *J Behav Med*. 2003;26:265–281.

13. Lackner JM, Gurtman MB. Pain catastrophizing and interpersonal problems: a circumplex analysis of the communal coping model. *Pain*. 2004;110:597–604.

14. Seminowicz DA, Davis KD. Cortical responses to pain in healthy individuals depends on pain catastrophizing. *Pain*. 2006;120:297–306.

15. Turk DC, Winter F. *The Pain Survival Guide: How to Reclaim Your Life*. Washington, DC: American Psychological Association; 2005.

16. Starr TD, Rogak LJ, Kirsh KL, Passik SD. Psychological and psychosocial evaluation. In: Fishman SM, Ballantyne JC, Rathmell JP, eds. *Bonica's Management of Pain*. 4th ed. Philadelphia: Lippincott Williams & Wilkins; 2009:270-278.

17. Kerns RD, Turk DC, Rudy TE. The West Haven-Yale Multidimensional Pain Inventory (WHYMPI). *Pain*. 1985 Dec;23(4):345-356.

18. Miakowski C, Zimmer EF, Barrett KM, et al. Differences in patients' and family caregivers' perceptions of the pain experience influence patient and caregiver outcomes. *Pain*. 1997;72:217–226.

19. American Psychiatric Association. *Diagnostic and Statistical Manual of Mental Disorders*. 4th ed text-rev. Washington, DC: Author; 2000:739.

20. Dersh J, Polatin PB, Gatchel RJ. Chronic pain and psychopathology: research findings and theoretical considerations. *Psychosom Med*. 2002 Sep-Oct;64(5):773-786.

21. Wasan AD, Sullivan MD, Clark MR. Psychiatric illness, depression, anxiety, and somatoform pain disorders. In Fishman SM, Ballantyne JC, Rathmell JP, eds. *Bonica's Management of Pain*. 4th ed. Philadelphia: Lippincott Williams & Wilkins; 2009:393-417.

22. Massie MJ. Prevalence of depression in patients with cancer. *J Natl Cancer Inst Monogr*. 2004;32:57–71.

23. Arnow BA, Hunkeler EM, Blasey CM, et al. Comorbid depression, chronic pain, and disability in primary care. *Psychosom Med*. 2006;68:262–268.

24. Pilowsky I. The diagnosis of abnormal illness behavior. *Aust N Z J Psychiatry*. 1971;5:136–141.

V.

Types of Pain

ACUTE PAIN

Postoperative Pain

Postoperative pain is arguably the most commonly occurring model of an acute pain condition. Despite its high prevalence, postoperative pain continues to be a challenging condition to treat, even in the face of continuing advances in pain management. The Joint Commission has developed guidelines for pain management specifically to try to improve consistency and effectiveness of pain assessment and treatment. These guidelines make clear recommendations on not only the importance of treatment of pain in hospitalized patients, but also continued assessment and reassessment of patients to uphold quality of pain management. Yet, a 2003 national survey revealed that 80% of adults surveyed who had undergone major surgery reported pain that was moderate to severe despite treatment with analgesics.[1]

Acute postoperative pain is likely managed by the pain service, an anesthesiologist, or a surgeon, either individually, or collaboratively. Specific types of postoperative pain and their individual treatments fall beyond the scope of this manual.

In the event that the responsibility of postoperative pain management falls on the shoulders of the primary care practitioner, some basic steps and considerations should be kept in mind that can improve the likelihood of effective treatment:

- **Preoperative discussion** should take place with the patient (if possible) to increase awareness of expectations of pain and its management and to minimize stress.

- **Detailed knowledge of use of analgesics *before* surgery** if applicable is important to estimate analgesic needs.

- **Pre-emptive analgesic therapy** may actually decrease post-procedure requirements for analgesics:
  - Nonsteroidal anti-inflammatory drugs
  - Cyclooxygenase-2 (COX-2) inhibitors (highly used for preemptive therapy in the past are now only valuable in selected patients where the benefit is clear and the patients are appropriate candidates)
  - Local anesthetics by direct injection
  - Opioids

- **Multimodal analgesic techniques**—using more than one method of pain management at the same time (see list above) can reduce the amount of medications necessary to relieve pain and can minimize uncomfortable side effects of any given medication.

Adequate postoperative pain management is an integral part of medical care in the postoperative period. It has also been shown, that poorly treated postoperative pain is more likely to become chronic in nature. Additional benefits of effective postoperative pain management include the following:

- Improved patient comfort
- Improved patient satisfaction
- Decreased time to ambulation
- Decreased rates of surgical complications
  - Bowel motility
  - Thrombophlebitic episodes
  - Improved blood flow and wound healing
  - Improved lung mechanics and severity of atelectasis

- Decreased length of hospital stay (non-ambulatory patients)

- Decreased return to hospital rates (ambulatory patients)

- Decreased cost of care

- Improved patient outcomes

Acute Pain Management for the Patient on Chronic Opioid Therapy

Changes in attitude have occurred in recent years regarding the use of opioids for the treatment of both cancer-related and noncancer-related pain. Both primary care clinicians and pain specialists prescribe opioids to a greater number of patients and in doses appropriate to individual patient needs. As the number of patients with chronic pain who are treated with chronic opioid therapy increases, the special challenge of appropriately managing acute pain in this patient population is becoming more common. There are a number of different reasons why chronic pain patients may experience acute pain: accident or injury-related pain, dental pain, and pain associated with surgical procedures.

Peri-operative pain is one of the most challenging and common reasons for acute pain management in chronic pain patients receiving chronic opioid therapy. These patients may need to undergo surgical procedures related to their chronic pain condition, such as back surgery, joint replacement, and tumor resection. Some clinicians cautiously underestimate theoretical intravenous dose equivalencies in patients who have already required extremely high baseline doses of oral or transdermal opioids. Ironically, this may be especially relevant to patients recovering from surgical procedures performed to reduce their baseline chronic pain. In any setting where pain is poorly controlled, patients may suffer, and develop untoward emotional and cognitive responses that negatively affect behavior, rehabilitation, and ultimately decreased quality of life.[2]

If it is reasonable to consider that a significant percentage of opioid naïve patients are subject to some degree of under-treatment of postsurgical pain (where they still report moderate to severe pain despite treatment), then it is also reasonable to predict this may be *exaggerated* in opioid-experienced patients, resulting from diminished opioid analgesic effectiveness. Tolerance may likely be an important contributor to this phenomenon.[3] **Analgesic tolerance** is defined as *decreasing analgesic effect* during long-term application of opioids, necessitating dose increases. Additionally, other mitigating factors may be involved as well, such as risk of withdrawal, physical or psychological dependence, or substance abuse. These concerns may be substantial, and may complicate clinical decisions about abrupt discontinuation or dose reduction.

Many patients who present for surgery and anesthesia may be opioid-dependent, or at least moderately tolerant to the therapeutic effects of opioid analgesics. Peri-operative management of opioid-experienced patients can present itself as a special challenge to primary caregivers, anesthesiologists, and pain specialists. This challenge mainly emanates from the conflicting need to balance the patient's analgesic needs and the concerns about addiction or dependency, and safety.

While there are no specific recommendations with regard to formulating a plan for managing acute pain, such as postoperative pain, in patients who are on chronic opioid therapy, there are general principles that should be considered a part of any treatment strategy:

- **Comprehension of concepts, terminology, and potential clinical impact:**
  - **Tolerance** (as defined above)
  - **Dependence**
    - Physical—actual alterations in physiologic response that result from opioid binding and receptor-mediated activity. May result in withdrawal signs and symptoms, such as hypertension, tachycardia, diaphoresis, and shaking.
    - Psychological—the perception that a substance causes a sense of well-being. May result in psychological-related signs and symptoms, such as depression or anxiety.

- **Awareness of behaviors related to substance abuse and misuse:**
  - **Addiction**
  - **Medication-seeking behavior**
  - **Pseudoaddiction**—a patient's attempt to compensate for development of tolerance, progression of disease, or worsening of pain. In general, pseudoaddictive patients can be differentiated from true drug abusers because increasing doses of opioids and improvement in pain control usually eliminate the drug-seeking behavior.
  - **Poor compliance**
- **A standardized peri-operative assessment strategy—** _**considered to be the most important step**_:
  - **Current medical regimen**   Patients may not know that opioids have been prescribed to them or may not recognize that escalations in their daily need for pain relievers reflects the development of tolerance.
  - **Abuse vs. use**   It is very important to distinguish between the two situations; while it is important to detect abusers, it is critically important to not falsely label patients who require opioids for analgesic efficacy as addicts.
  - **Tolerance vs. dependence**   It is necessary to develop a clear management strategy that maintains a balance of gaining patient trust with an understanding and caring approach, while being prepared to overcome high-grade tolerance with liberal doses of opioid _**and nonopioid analgesics**_, as part of a multimodal treatment plan.
  - **Substance abuse history**   It is important to consider the fact that patients with substance use disorders involving licit or illicit substances (e.g., alcohol, marijuana, cocaine, heroin, or nicotine) show a higher incidence of dependence on other substances than the general population.[4]

- **Treatment plan formulation and patient expectations** Knowledge of the surgical procedure, the likely degree of postoperative pain, and the context of the patient's postoperative location (such as ambulatory vs. hospitalization).

■ **A standardized approach to peri-operative opioid use:**

- Continuation of currently prescribed analgesic opioids up to the day of surgery
- *Pre-operative administration* of their daily maintenance dose prior to anesthetic induction
- Maintenance of existing baseline opioid requirements, orally if the patient is ambulatory, and by Patient Controlled Analgesia (PCA) for inpatients
- Continuation of maintenance medications (e.g., methadone) for recovering addicted patients
- Consideration that opioid doses required to meet postsurgical analgesic requirements are affected by receptor down-regulation and may need to be increased 30-100%, in comparison with requirements in opioid-naïve patients[5]
- Consideration of the fact that there are differences in oral to intravenous dose equivalency, which need to be appreciated to estimate peri-operative baseline and supplemental opioid dose requirements; parenteral administration bypasses gastrointestinal absorption variables and first-pass hepatic clearance and metabolism

Although it may be a part of the long-term clinical plan, it is worth pointing out that when a patient is experiencing acute pain, such as postoperative pain, *is not the time to attempt detoxification or rehabilitation*.

It is also important to keep in mind that non-opioid analgesic adjuvants, such as non-steroidal anti-inflammatory agents, local anesthetics, anti-convulsants, and other agents, may also be used to reduce opioid dose requirements and provide multimodal analgesia.

Fear and anxiety can also contribute to the pain experience. These should be discussed with the patient and treated with appropriate therapies as necessary. The major consideration is to avoid under-medicating patients with acute pain with careful titration, standardization of practice, and most of all, safety. Awareness and administration of appropriate doses of analgesics as well as continuous clinical monitoring remain the keys to successful peri-operative pain management in this group of patients.[2]

CHRONIC PAIN

Back and Neck Pain

The structural framework of the neck and back consist of the vertebrae, musculature, and ligaments. As already stated, the likelihood is that four out of five people will experience some type of back pain in their lives.[6] The epidemiology of neck and back pain is vast. Back pain is also one of the most common forms of chronic pain in patients at all age ranges.[7] Low back pain (LBP) is well-distributed across sex, race, and marital status,[8] and it is among the top 10 complaints of patients older than 16 years of age who present to the primary care practitioner,[9] with a prevalence of up to 20%.[10] Although neck pain often receives less publicity than LBP, millions of people experience neck pain and/or related arm pain at some point in their lives.

The economic and social magnitude of the impact of neck and back pain—most frequently chronic LBP—is enormous. Although it is difficult to calculate exactly how much back pain costs in the United States, statistics show that backaches result in the loss of approximately 175 million work days and in a $20 billion dollar loss in productivity. Two percent of the U.S. work force suffers from chronic back pain, costing the U.S. economy a total of $50 billion dollars annually. The general complaint of backache is the second most common reason Americans seek medical attention (headaches are the first), and among the most common reasons for surgery (National Institutes of Health data on file).[11]

Temporal Classification of Back and Neck Pain

Acute back or neck pain generally arises spontaneously and usually lasts from a few days to a few months. Such pain may or may not have radicular symptoms associated with it. Treatment for acute back and neck pain is usually symptomatic and typically includes activity as tolerated and some form of analgesia. Bed rest for more than 2 days has now been shown conclusively to worsen prognosis. In fact, the debunking of the myth that rest is helpful, with the consequent reduction of iatrogenic disability, is probably the major advance in the treatment of back pain in the modern era.[12]

Persistent, or *chronic*, back or neck pain may be defined as pain that lasts 3-6 months, or longer, and does not improve over time. In cases of chronic back pain, there is a high correlation with spondylotic disease. Patients with persistent pain often undergo surgical intervention,[6] although results are inconsistent. It has been recently appreciated that many patients have neither acute back pain nor chronic persistent back pain, but instead have recurrent back pain, or constant back trouble that occasionally becomes severe and disabling. These patients may experience long-term difficulties, including psychological and medical comorbidities. Some common psychological problems include depression, anxiety, and sleep disturbance.

Multidisciplinary interventions, emphasizing rehabilitation, are commonly required.

Common *pathologic* causes of back and neck pain include the following:

- Disc herniation
- Sciatica
- Torticollis
- Spinal stenosis
- Spondylosis
- Spondylolisthesis
- Cauda equina syndrome
- Cancer
- Primary tumor

- Metastatic lesion
- Osteomyelitis of the spine
- Injury (e.g., fracture, compression)
- As a direct result of trauma
- As a result of osteoporotic disease

Making the diagnosis in cases of chronic back and neck pain can be challenging for primary caregivers and experts. Although diagnostic procedures have continued to improve in their accuracy and reliability, up to 85% of chronic cases may end up with no definitive diagnosis.[13] Sometimes the identifiable causes are muscular, but in the face of accompanying neurologic deficit, there may indeed be some degree of neurologic etiology. Although sometimes episodes of back and neck pain have no identifiable anatomic cause, there are many cases where this pain can be linked to a known cause, such as the following:

- Overuse, strenuous activity, or improper use, such as repetitive or heavy lifting
- Muscle injury
  - Strain
  - Torticollis
- Whiplash (sudden force injury)
- Concurrent diagnosis of cancer
- Trauma
  - Injury/contusion
  - Fracture
- Degeneration of vertebrae, often caused by stresses on the muscles and ligaments that support the spine, or the effects of aging
- Infection
- Abnormal growth, such as a tumor or bone spur
- Obesity with the result of increased weight on the spine and pressure on the disks
- Poor muscle tone

- Muscle tension or spasm
- Ligament or muscle tears
- Joint problems, such as arthritis
- Protruding or herniated disk and/or nerve impingement
- Osteoporosis and compression fractures
- Congenital/developmental abnormalities of the vertebrae and bones (i.e., scoliosis)

Evaluation of Low Back Pain

Low back pain is the fifth most common reason for all medical visits in the United States,[14] and although there are many recommendations that are available for evaluation and management of low back pain, there has been a lack of consensus for consistency in evaluation in the past. Like any other painful condition, the assessment of LBP should begin with a detailed history of the pain, including the patient's perception of its cause and the location and duration of the pain. A careful history is necessary to formulate diagnostic impressions and determine what the cause of the pain is.

The most important goal in assessing the patient with LBP is to *rule out 'diagnostic imperatives', that is, serious illnesses that can present with LBP.* These include dissecting aortic aneurysm, cancer or infections involving the spine, inflammatory spondylitis, and referred pain from the abdominal or pelvic viscera. Factors that suggest the need to rule out such disorders include new-onset back pain in an older patient, systemic symptoms (e.g., fever, sweats, and weight loss), history of cancer, and abdominal or pelvic pain.

During the physical examination, observe the patient's gait and overall posture. Scoliosis may point to underlying muscle spasm or neurogenic involvement. The examiner should also test the patient's spinal range of motion. Although the reliability of provocative maneuvers is not high, reproduction of pain on lumbar flexion tends to indicate disc pathology; pain on extension suggests facet joint pathology. The examiner should also palpate the spine for point tenderness, which could help determine the site of pathology. Palpation of the abdomen and pelvis and examination for signs of systemic illness are imperative in the evaluation of all patients with acute or subacute LBP, especially with the risk factors noted above. Suspicion of lumbosacral radiculopathy, suggested by radiating pain or by accompanying neurologic symptoms, can be confirmed with provocative maneuvers. In the straight leg raise test, pain radiating below the knee when the leg is raised between 30 and 60 degrees suggests nerve root irritation. The straight-leg raise test is used as a test for sciatica, the lay term for *lumbosacral radiculopathy*. The crossed straight leg raise test, which tests/assesses for pain radiating down the contralateral leg when the ipsilateral leg is raised, is a less sensitive, but highly specific test for lumbosacral radiculopathy.[15] A focused neurologic examination should be performed. More details can be found in Chapter IV. Reflexes (knee and ankle) and motor and sensory testing should also be conducted to determine the presence of a neurologic deficit, which could indicate lumbosacral radiculopathy, cauda equina syndrome, or even spinal cord involvement.

Laboratory tests are not usually needed during an initial evaluation of LBP. However, if risk factors suggest tumor or infection, appropriate blood work and imaging studies must be obtained.

In October 2007, a new set of clinical guidelines were published jointly by the American Pain Society (APS), and the American College of Physicians (ACP),[16] to bring some consistency to the processes of evaluation and management of low back pain. These guidelines are intended to present the available evidence for standardized evaluation and management of acute and chronic low back pain in primary care settings. The target audience for these guidelines is *"all clinicians caring for patients with low (lumbar) back pain of any duration, either with or without leg pain. The target patient populations are adults with acute and chronic low back pain not associated with major trauma, children or adolescents with low back pain, and pregnant women; patients with low back pain from other sources (non-spinal low back pain), fibromyalgia or other myofascial pain syndromes, and thoracic or cervical back pain, are also included."*

The ACP/APS guidelines make the following specific recommendations for the evaluation of low back pain:

1. Clinicians should conduct a **focused history and physical examination** to help place patients with low back pain into one of three broad categories:
   a. Nonspecific back pain
   b. Back pain potentially associated with radiculopathy or spinal stenosis
   c. Back pain potentially associated with another specific spinal cause

The history should include assessment of psychosocial risk factors, which predict risk for chronic disabling back pain.

2. Clinicians should *not* **routinely obtain imaging or other diagnostic tests** in patients with nonspecific low back pain.

3. Clinicians *should* **perform diagnostic imaging and testing** for patients with low back pain when severe or progressive neurologic deficits are present, or when serious underlying conditions are suspected on the basis of history and physical examination.

4. Clinicians *should* evaluate patients with persistent low back pain and signs or symptoms of radiculopathy or spinal stenosis with magnetic resonance imaging (preferred), or computerized tomography, **only if they are potential candidates for surgery or epidural steroid injection** (for suspected radiculopathy).

Treatment of Low Back Pain

Because the progression of low back pain from acute to chronic is a major problem, it is worth keeping in mind strategies targeted towards preventing this progression. Other major risks for chronicity are psychosocial: comorbid psychiatric disorders, previous disabling episodes, and poor job satisfaction. It is advisable to perform a psychosocial assessment screening on patients with acute low back pain so that high-risk patients can be promptly referred for multidisciplinary rehabilitative management, with vocational rehabilitation if needed.

The ACP/APS Clinical Practice Guidelines recommend the following with respect to the treatment of low back pain:

1. Clinicians should **provide patients with evidence-based information** on low back pain with regard to their expected course, advise patients to remain active, and provide information about effective self-care options.

2. For patients with low back pain, clinicians should **consider the use of medications with proven benefits in conjunction with back care information and self-care**. Clinicians should assess severity of baseline pain and functional deficits, potential benefits, risks, and relative lack of long-term efficacy and safety data before initiating therapy. For most patients, first-line medication options are acetaminophen or nonsteroidal anti-inflammatory drugs.

3. **For patients who do not improve with self-care options, clinicians should consider the addition of nonpharmacologic therapy with proven benefits**—for acute low back pain, spinal manipulation; for chronic or subacute low back pain, intensive interdisciplinary rehabilitation, exercise therapy, acupuncture, massage therapy, spinal manipulation, yoga, cognitive-behavioral therapy, or progressive relaxation.

■ **Table 5.1**
Pharmacologic Treatment of Back and Neck Pain

Once the diagnostic imperatives have been ruled out, treatment is symptomatic and is directed toward providing pain relief and restoring function.

- ■ Most patients benefit from **maintenance of activity as tolerated, keeping as active as they can**.
- ■ This process is often best directed by a physical therapist.

Nonsteroidal anti-inflammatory drugs are helpful for acute low back pain, given the potential risks outlined in Chapter VI.

A short course of **opioid analgesics** is often required, although it is easy to overestimate their efficacy.

- ■ A patient who cannot stand up due to acute low back pain may not stand much better while taking opioids. However, opioids can facilitate more comfortable rest periods and can facilitate reintroduction of activity and exercise.

(continued)

■ **Table 5.1**
  Pharmacologic Treatment of Back and Neck Pain *(continued)*

Muscle relaxants are frequently prescribed for acute low back pain and probably have analgesic efficacy, although they do not have any primary effect on muscles. Although clinicians attempting to avoid opioid use often prescribe muscle relaxants, little is accomplished for the patient by this approach because the muscle relaxants share most of the liabilities of the opioids.

The benefits of **nonpharmacologic approaches** should not be underestimated—a well-constructed comparative trial has shown that a heating pad provided more analgesia than a nonsteroidal anti-inflammatory drug.[13]

Many practitioners perform **epidural steroid injections** on patients with acute sciatica to reduce nerve inflammation and prevent chronicity, although this approach has never been validated.

■**Oral steroids are generally *not* indicated** for the treatment of back and neck pain.

Antidepressants have been widely used for both depressed and non-depressed patients with chronic low back problems. The extent to which these medications are used in treating patients with acute low back problems is unknown. Some researchers have hypothesized that the medications may possibly have a pain-relieving effect in addition to antidepressant properties. If so, the medications could help some patients who have chronic pain whether or not the patients are also depressed. The therapeutic objective of using antidepressant medications for low back problems is to reduce pain (See more discussion of antidepressants in Chapter VI.)

Because the progression of low back pain from acute to chronic is a major problem, it is worth keeping in mind strategies for prevention of this progression. The major risks for chronicity are psychosocial: comorbid psychiatric disorders, previous disabling episodes, poor job satisfaction, and so forth. It is advisable to perform a psychosocial assessment screening on patients with acute low back pain so that high-risk patients can be promptly referred for multidisciplinary rehabilitative management, with vocational rehabilitation if needed.

Headache

The most common of all pain syndromes is headache. As stated previously, studies show that the large majority of adults experience headaches and that headache pain is the single largest factor in work absenteeism, as well as total expenditures for health care costs.

Headaches are usually characterized by attacks that are separated by symptom-free intervals, but sometimes may become chronic. Headaches can be caused by structural abnormalities, sinus disease, increased intracranial pressure, or even referred pain from the cervical spine.

The following are three major hypotheses concerning the various origins of headache:

1. Neurogenic or vascular abnormalities in the brain

2. Myofascial or skeletal mechanisms from the cervical spine

3. A variety of diseases involving the face

The ability to make a rapid and accurate diagnosis is crucial to the successful management of any headache disorder. Because head pain can have many causes, a rational approach facilitates differential diagnosis and may increase the likelihood of a positive therapeutic outcome.

Classification of Headaches

Headaches are commonly classified as either primary or secondary. The *primary* headache disorders—those *not* associated with an underlying pathology—include migraine, tension-type, and cluster headaches. *Secondary headache* disorders—those attributed to an underlying pathologic condition—include any head pain of infectious, neoplastic, vascular, drug-induced, or idiopathic origin. The vast majority of patients who present with headache have one of the primary disorders, as serious secondary causes for presentation with head pain are rare.

A number of diagnostic schemata for headache have been proposed. As early as 1962, for example, the Ad Hoc Committee on Classification of Headache listed the features that are typically present during certain types of headaches, but it failed to indicate which features or combinations of features were required to establish a diagnosis. By 1988, recognizing the need for improvement in headache classification, the *International Headache Society* (IHS) published a new system, the second edition of the International Headache Classification (ICHD-2).

The following information is based on and adapted from the updated IHS criteria, ICHD-2, which outline the classification, incidence, prevalence, and specific characteristics necessary to confirm a broad range of headache disorders.[17]

Primary Headache

Migraine Headache. Migraine is a chronic neurologic disorder characterized by episodic attacks of head pain and associated symptoms. Similar epidemiologic studies conducted 10 years apart show that the prevalence and distribution of migraine have remained stable over the last decade in the United States, with approximately 18% of women and 6% of men satisfying diagnostic criteria for the condition. Studies conducted outside the United States are in agreement with these migraine prevalence rates. Even though it is widespread, migraine often remains under-diagnosed; only 48% of Americans who satisfy criteria for migraine reported receiving a physician diagnosis of migraine. Many patients *(estimated to be approximately 50%)* never even seek medical advice and treat themselves with over-the-counter medications for this condition. The IHS recognizes six variants of migraine, but the most common types seen in primary care practice are migraine with aura (formerly "classic" migraine), migraine without aura (formerly "common" migraine), and probable migraine (formerly "migrainous headache").

Migraine with Aura. Providers should suspect migraine with aura whenever a headache is preceded by one of the neurologic symptoms listed in Table 5.2.

The symptoms of migraine with aura should be reported as fully reversible, developing over 5–20 minutes and lasting less than 60 minutes. It is commonly observed in clinical practice that not all auras are followed by a headache or a headache that is associated with characteristics of migraine. If aura occurs without subsequent

■ **Table 5.2**
Adapted International Headache Society Criteria for Migraine

Migraine with Aura	Migraine without Aura* (At Least Any Two Descriptions)	Migraine without Aura* (At Least Any One Symptom)
Visual symptoms	Unilateral nature	Nausea and/or
Blind spots	Pulsatile quality	vomiting
Flashes of light	of pain	Photophobia
"Zigzag" light	Moderate	Phonophobia
Other visual	to severe	
distortions	intensity	
Motor Weakness	Aggravation by,	
Sensory Symptoms	or causing	
Parasthesia	avoidance of	
Aphasia	routine physical	
Signs of brain stem	activity	
dysfunction		
Diplopia		
Ataxia		
Vertigo		

*Patients without aura must have five attacks fulfilling the above criteria, with headaches lasting 4–72 hrs, and no signs of a secondary headache disorder, to meet criteria.

headache, then the condition is a typical aura without headache; if a non-migraine headache follows aura, then it is classified as a typical aura with a non-migraine headache.

Migraine without Aura. Migraine without aura is the commonest subtype of migraine. It has a higher average attack frequency and is usually more disabling than migraine with aura. Migraine without aura is characterized by headache pain that is virtually indistinguishable from the pain experienced by patients with aura, except no aura precedes the migraine attack.

Migraine without aura is often thought to have a strict menstrual relationship. In contrast to the first edition of *The International*

Classification of Headache Disorders, the current edition gives criteria for *pure menstrual migraine* and *menstrually related migraine* in the appendix, because of uncertainty over whether they should be regarded as separate entities. Because of their frequency, and menstrual relationship, they deserve mention. *(www.PainEDU.org has more detailed information on migraine headaches and their menstrual relationship.)*

Pure Menstrual Migraine. Pure menstrual migraine has the following distinguishing characteristics:

- Attacks in a menstruating woman

- Fulfilling criteria for migraine without aura

- Attacks occur exclusively on day 1±2 (i.e., days –2 to +3) of menstruation in at least two out of three menstrual cycles and at *no other times of the cycle*

Menstrually Related Migraine. Menstrually related migraine has the following distinguishing characteristics:

- Attacks in a menstruating woman

- Fulfilling criteria for migraine without aura

- Attacks occur on day 1±2 (i.e., days –2 to +3) of menstruation in at least two out of three menstrual cycles and *in addition at other times of the cycle*

Because migraine without aura does not have a single distinguishing feature, the IHS criteria for migraine without aura require the presence of a constellation of symptoms (see Table 5.2).

Despite the existence of specific criteria of both types of migraine, clinicians frequently misdiagnose migraine. One reason for error is the criteria themselves. The IHS criteria do not include all symptoms frequently observed in episodes of migraine. Consequently, migraine associated with muscle or neck pain, a non-IHS migraine diagnostic criterion, is often diagnosed as tension-type headache (TTH), or migraine associated with nasal symptoms such as rhinorrhea and nasal congestion, also not included as IHS diagnostic criteria, is diagnosed

■ **Table 5.3**
Treatment of Migraine Headache Pain

1. Treatment should be adapted to the patient's individual needs, in view of his or her medical history and mental health.

2. Migraine treatment strategies are often considered to be one of two approaches:

   a. **Abortive treatment** (getting rid of an acute headache)

   b. **Prophylactic treatment** (preventing headaches)

3. First, **precipitating factors should be identified** so that the patient can learn to **avoid them**, if possible. These factors include the following:

   a. Alcohol

   b. Abrupt changes in climate or weather

   c. Diet

   d. Missing meals

   e. Stress

   f. Hormonal changes (including menstruation, ovulation, and menopause)

   g. Lack of sleep

4. **Teaching** the patient coping skills is also helpful.

5. **With regard to acute measures, all of the treatment strategies are more effective when combined with treating coexisting insomnia.**

6. **Nonsteroidal anti-inflammatory drugs** or **high doses of aspirin** are effective in treating migraine.[18] However, the gastrointestinal side effects of such medications may require that they be administered through the rectal or parenteral route. Moreover, an antiemetic may be needed to counteract the effects of treatment.

7. **Serotonin (5-HT) agonists** (e.g., triptans such as sumatriptan, rizatriptan, and zolmitriptan) are the most effective drugs for aborting a migraine episode. **Sumatriptan** is the most commonly prescribed triptan; however, it also has many side effects. Triptans are contraindicated for patients with

(continued)

■ **Table 5.3**
  Treatment of Migraine Headache Pain *(continued)*

---

cardiovascular or cerebrovascular disorders because of their vasoconstrictive action.

8. Other options for acute treatment of migraine include **antiemetics** and **intranasal dihydroergotamine**.

9. Although **ergotamine** treatments were commonly used to treat migraines in the past, they are generally used only for headaches that have been resistant to other treatments.[19]

10. Prophylactic treatments of migraine are usually considered in cases where the patient's migraines are frequent and disabling, a common rule being more than three severe headaches per month. Research indicates that the long-term efficacy of prophylactic measures is only about 55%.

    a. Prophylactic treatment may also be beneficial in cases of menstrually-related migraines, with drugs such as **frovatriptan**.

    b. Other drugs found effective for preventing migraines may be considered despite the occurrence of side effects that may make them more or less reasonable for a given patient, include the following:

        i. **Beta blockers**

        ii. **Sodium valproate**

        iii. **Gabapentin**

        iv. **Serotonin antagonists**

        v. **Calcium channel blockers**

    c. Nonpharmacologic treatments, including **biofeedback**, **behavioral therapy**, and **acupuncture**, are also effective in preventing migraine headaches.[18,19]

---

as a "sinus" headache. In both cases, research demonstrates that these headaches are usually migraine. Additionally, clinicians often focus on the presence of a single symptom to make a migraine diagnosis. This often results in even experts having different opinions of whether or not a headache is truly a migraine.

An especially significant complicating factor in the diagnosis of migraine may be the existence of comorbid illness. Migraine has also been associated with a number of psychiatric and medical-neurologic illnesses. Therefore, providers should not be surprised to find an increased incidence of affective and anxiety disorders among migraine patients. Bipolar psychiatric disturbances and phobias are also noted. The incidence of stroke, epilepsy, essential tremor, mitral valve prolapse, and Raynaud's disease also are increased in migraine patients compared with their non-migraine counterparts. (*www.PainEDU.org has more detailed information on migraine headaches.*)

Tension-Type Headache. TTH is the **most common** type of primary headache. In the general population, estimates by the IHS of the prevalence of episodic TTH vary widely, from 30 to 80%. The IHS criteria for TTH, listed in Table 5.4, outline a range of specific characteristics that distinguish TTH from migraine and show that the symptoms tend to be less severe, bilateral, non-pulsating, and not aggravated by routine physical activity. Symptoms associated with migraine attacks, such as nausea, phonophobia, or photophobia, are rarely present, but there can be symptomatic overlap. Studies have shown that 25% of TTH patients also have migraine, and 62% of migraineurs have TTH. Moreover, epidemiologic research suggests that TTH, when it coexists with migraine, might represent a segment on the continuum of the same disorder.

In the 2004 IHS diagnostic criteria, episodic TTH, as opposed to chronic daily TTH, is a condition without associated symptoms other than photophobia or phonophobia. Although this further separates migraine and tension headache, it leaves more headache presentations of a mixed type. Much of the void is filled by a diagnosis of "probable migraine," which represents a headache that lacks one diagnostic criterion for migraine headache.

■ **Table 5.4**
   Adapted International Headache Society
   Criteria for Tension-Type Headache*

Description (At Least Any Two Descriptions)	Associated Symptoms (At Least One)
Pressing or tightening	Absence of nausea or vomiting
Mild to moderate intensity	Photophobia *or* phonophobia
Bilateral location	(not both)
No worsening with exertion	

*Must have had more than 10 previous headache episodes and no evidence of a secondary headache disorder

■ **Table 5.5**
   Treatment of Tension-Type Headache Pain

1. Research shows that **nonsteroidal anti-inflammatory drugs** are the primary treatment of choice for acute tension-type headaches.[19]

2. **Combining analgesics with caffeine or sedatives** may be more effective than analgesics alone.

3. **There is no scientific evidence that muscle relaxants are an effective treatment.**

4. Tricyclic antidepressants are often prescribed as prophylactic treatment for chronic tension-type headaches. **Amitriptyline** is the most frequently prescribed antidepressant, but it has many side effects. When the patient experiences these side effects, some other antidepressants, such as **nortriptyline** or **desipramine**, can be used.

5. **Cognitive-behavioral strategies** are also effective for reducing stress, and research shows that these strategies are most effective when combined with **biofeedback or relaxation techniques**.

6. Some other nonpharmacologic treatments include **massage, positioning, and heat or cold applications**.

Cluster Headache. Cluster headaches are the third major type of primary headache and are defined as a strictly unilateral headache, usually occurring once or a few times a day at a characteristic time (e.g., 1 a.m.), lasting for 15–180 minutes, occurring in a series which lasts from several weeks to several months, separated by remissions lasting from months to years.

Findings from prevalence studies of cluster headache are controversial. Patients with cluster headaches generally rate the intensity of their pain as among the worst imaginable, and cluster headache may be the most severe of the primary headache disorders. Most often, cluster headache occurs once every 24 hours for 6–12 weeks at a time, with remission periods typically lasting 12 months. Typical age of onset for both men and women is 27–31 years. However, **cluster headaches are one of the few headache syndromes that are more frequent in men than in women.** Population studies of cluster headaches find the occurrence is five times more likely in males. Cluster headaches may be related to cigarette smoking, head trauma, and positive family history for cluster headaches.

Cluster attacks have several differentiating features. Most important of these is the presence of transient autonomic symptoms.

These features are listed in Table 5.6

■ **Table 5.6**
Adapted International Headache Society Criteria for Cluster Headache*

Description (All Four Descriptions)	Autonomic Symptoms (Any Two Symptoms)
Severe headache	Rhinorrhea
Unilateral and ipsilateral quality	Lacrimation
Duration of 15–180 mins	Facial sweating
Orbital, periorbital, or	Miosis
temporal location	Eyelid edema
	Conjunctival injection
	Ptosis

*No evidence of a secondary headache disorder

■ **Table 5.7**
  Treatment of Cluster Headache Pain

---

1. **In most cases, patients with cluster headaches should be referred to a specialist.**

2. Acute treatment of cluster headaches includes the following:

   a. Inhalation of **100% oxygen**

   b. Intranasal application of **dihydroergotamine**

   c. Subcutaneous injection of **sumatriptan**

3. There is no *consensus as to prophylactic treatment* of cluster headaches. Some methods include prescribing the following:

   a. **Verapamil**

   b. **Lithium carbonate**

   c. **Methysergide**

   d. **Ergotamine**

   e. **Corticosteroids**

Systemic symptoms, such as bradycardia, hypertension, and increased gastric acid production, may also accompany an attack. Another unique feature is that cluster episodes are always on the same side, even when long intervals separate headache episodes.

Diagnosis of Primary Headache in Clinical Practice

Because most office-based evaluations of headache occur when patients are asymptomatic, the primary health care provider relies on *impact-based recognition* of headache. On those occasions when a person is being evaluated during a headache, it is best to rely on IHS criteria, summarized in Table 5.8.[17]

■ **Table 5.8**
Characteristics of Primary Headache Disorders

	Migraine	Tension-Type	Cluster
Location	Unilateral	Bilateral	Strictly unilateral
Intensity	Moderate/severe	Mild/moderate	Severe
Duration	4–72 hours	30 mins to 7 days	15–90 mins
Quality	Throbbing	Pressing/tightening	Severe
Associated Symptoms	Yes	No	Yes, autonomic
Gender	Female> Male	Female > Male	Male > Female

Given the constraints of clinical practice, however, primary headache disorders can be quickly and reliably recognized by inquiring about the following:

■ Interference with daily living

■ Recurrent disabling headaches should be considered migraine until proven otherwise

■ Frequency

  ■ The frequency of headaches alerts the clinician to chronic headache disorders and migraine transformation

  ■ Daily or near-daily headache patterns should alert the provider to the possibility of medication overuse

■ Change in headache pattern over prior 6-month period

  ■ A negative response reassures the caregiver and the patient that serious underlying disease is unlikely

  ■ An affirmative answer indicates the need for a more in depth evaluation of possible warning signs that a secondary headache disorder may be present

- Change in existing headaches
  - "Worst headache ever"
- Focal neurologic signs or symptoms such as the following:
  - Papilledema
  - Motor weakness
  - Memory loss
  - Papillary abnormalities
  - Sensory loss
- Association with systemic symptoms
- New-onset headache after age 50
- Medication use
  - More than 2 days a week
    - Overuse of any acute headache remedy, prescription or nonprescription, *may promote more frequent headaches*
    - "Medication-induced migraine"

Secondary Headache

As mentioned in "Classification of Headaches," secondary headache disorders are those **attributed to an underlying pathologic condition**. Obviously, the focus centers around the headache-causing condition when dealing with diagnosis.

The breakdown of conditions that cause secondary headache identified by the IHS are the following:

- Head and/or neck trauma
- Cranial or cervical vascular disorder
- Cranial nonvascular disorder
- A substance or its withdrawal
- Infection
- Disorder of the cranium, neck, eyes, ears, nose, sinuses, teeth, mouth, or other facial or cranial structure
- Psychiatric disorder

The following criteria should be used for assistance in diagnosis and distinguishing secondary from primary headache:

- Another disorder known to be able to cause headache has been demonstrated.

- Headache occurs in close temporal relation to the other disorder, and/or there is other evidence of a causal relationship.

- Headache is greatly reduced or resolves within 3 months (possibly shorter for some disorders) after successful treatment or spontaneous remission of the causative disorder.

Arthritis Pain

Based on 2003–2005 data from the National Health Interview Survey, 46 million American adults reported doctor-diagnosed arthritis, making arthritis one of the nation's most common health problems.[20] As a result of this, arthritis is very commonly seen in primary care practices. Obviously, as the U.S. population ages, these numbers are likely to increase dramatically. The number of people who have doctor-diagnosed arthritis is projected to increase to 67 million in 2030.[21]

Arthritis is actually not a single disease, but a constellation consisting of more than 100 different conditions. Among the most common are osteoarthritis (OA) and rheumatoid arthritis (RA). Considering the costs associated with diagnosis, treatment, and lost productivity due to disability, arthritis is one of the most expensive diseases in the United States today.[20] Arthritis is actually *the nation's leading cause of disability*, limiting everyday activities for 19 million Americans in 2005.[20] Work limitations attributable to arthritis affect more than 5% of the general population and over 30% of people with arthritis.[20] Each year, arthritis results in 750,000 hospitalizations and 36 million outpatient visits. Direct medical costs for arthritis were more than $80 billion in 2003.[22] Arthritis is not just an old person's disease. Nearly two-thirds of people with arthritis are younger than age 65.[20]

Osteoarthritis

OA is the most common arthritic condition, affecting an estimated 27 million Americans, usually 60 years of age or older.[23] OA is primarily a disease of the cartilage that results in local tissue response, mechanical change, and, ultimately, failure of function.

The joints most commonly involved in presentation of OA typically include the following:

- Cervical spine
- Distal interphalangeal joints
- Feet and ankles
- First carpometacarpal joints
- Hips
- Knees
- Lower spine
- Proximal interphalangeal joints

Patients usually present with symptoms of *morning stiffness lasting no longer than 20–30 minutes*. Presence of stiffness that persists longer should generate inquiry about other possible diagnoses. In the absence of injury, involvement of the shoulders, wrists, and elbows is uncommon.

Diagnosis of OA is assisted by attention to the following:

- Clinical presentation
  - History and physical findings
- Radiographic evaluation
  - Joint space narrowing of large, weight bearing joints
  - Increased subchondral bony sclerosis
  - Osteophytes
  - Small synovial effusions with noninflammatory pathology findings
  - Laboratory tests are usually not useful and often normal

2008 OARSI Management Guidelines for Osteoarthritis of Hip and Knee

The Osteoarthritis Research Society International (OARSI) recently published a set of guidelines[24] for management of patients with osteoarthritis. The OARSI convened a group of sixteen international experts from a variety of medical disciplines, including primary care, rheumatology, and orthopedics, with the goal of developing a set of rational, evidenced-based guidelines for the management of osteoarthritis (OA) of the hip and knee.

The purpose of these guidelines are to *"provide concise, patient focused, up to date, evidence-based, expert consensus recommendations for the management of hip and knee OA, which are globally relevant"* to physicians and allied health care professionals who manage OA in both primary care and expert practice settings. They also take into account that there may be regional variations in availability of some treatment approaches.

The development process involved a systematic review of existing guidelines for the management of hip and knee OA published between 1945 and January 2006, and a core set of management modalities was generated based on the agreement between guidelines. Evidence before 2002 was based on a systematic review conducted by European League Against Rheumatism and evidence after 2002 was updated using MEDLINE, EMBASE, CINAHL, AMED, The Cochrane Library, and HTA reports.

After rigorous review, the following recommendations were made within the context of the four major categories of treatment:

General

- A management plan that utilizes a combination of pharmacologic and non- pharmacologic modalities, with the intention of curbing disease progress, managing pain, and improving quality of life.

Nonpharmacologic

- Information access and patient education about:
  - The objectives of treatment
  - Pacing of activities

- Necessary changes in lifestyle (e.g., exercise, weight reduction)
- Compliance to therapy
- Self-help and patient-driven treatments

■ Regular contact (e.g., by phone) to assess status

■ Physical therapy and muscle strengthening

■ Encouragement for overweight patients to lose weight, and maintain weight loss

■ Use of mobility aids, such as a cane, crutch, or walker

■ Bracing when appropriate to reduce pain, improve stability, and diminish fall risk

■ Appropriate footwear

■ Complementary techniques including:
  - Thermal applications
  - Transcutaneous electronic nerve stimulation (TENS)
  - Acupuncture

Pharmacologic

■ Acetaminophen (up to 4 gm/day) for initial analgesic treatment of mild to moderate pain

■ Non-steroidal anti-inflammatory drugs (NSAIDS) at the lowest effective dose, avoiding long-term use if possible*

■ Topical NSAIDS or capsaicin as alternatives or adjuncts to analgesic therapy

■ Intra-articular injections:
  - Corticosteroids, particularly when there is refractory pain or distinct signs of local inflammation
  - Hyaluaronate may also be useful, but may take a reasonable amount of time to demonstrate efficacy

---

*In patients with increased GI risk, a COX-2 selective agent, or a non-selective NSAID with co-prescription of a proton pump inhibitor (PPI), for gastroprotection may be considered. NSAIDs, including both non-selective and COX-2 selective agents, should always be used with caution in patients with cardiovascular risk factors.

Opioids for the treatment of refractory pain with the above-mentioned treatments, along with consideration of surgical intervention

Surgical

- Joint replacement arthroplasties are effective, and cost-effective, interventions for patients with significant symptoms and/or functional limitations; these limitations are associated with a reduced health-related quality of life, despite conservative therapy.

These are core recommendations for the treatment of OA of the hip and knee. It is anticipated that over time they will need to be adapted, and possibly modified; the OARSI plans to monitor research evidence annually, and to update the guidelines every 3–5 years as necessary.

Rheumatoid Arthritis

RA is the second most common form of arthritis. It is a debilitating and destructive disease and, unlike OA, a systemic inflammatory condition. Women are affected more than men (5:1). Incidence is highest between ages 20 and 50, with a prevalence of 1–2% of adults, ranging from 0.3% in patients younger than 35 to approximately 10% of those older than 65 years old.[25]

RA is a chronic autoimmune disease; patients present with findings including the following:

- Symmetric involvement of small and large joints with the following:
  - Pain
  - Swelling
  - Warmth
  - Tenderness
  - Synovitis
  - Occurs in patients typically younger than OA patients
  - Morning stiffness lasts several hours to entire day
  - Fever
  - Weight loss

Diagnosis of RA is assisted by attention to the following clinical presentation:

- History and physical findings
  - Chronic progressive system inflammation
    - Joint swelling
    - Synovitis
- Large joint effusions
- Pathology positive for the following:
  - Elevated white blood cell count (20,000–50,000) with 50–70% polymorphonuclear leukocyte cells
- Laboratory tests
  - Elevated erythrocyte sedimentation rate
  - Elevated C-reactive protein
  - Anemia of chronic disease
  - Rheumatoid factor present in 90% of patients
- Radiographic studies
  - Juxtaarticular osteoporosis may be present
  - Symmetric affectation

In addition to the structural and mechanical consequences of arthritis, pain is a significant stress for people with the condition. People with OA and RA experience both acute and chronic pain, depending on the progression of their condition. A major consideration in dealing with arthritis patients is the patient's level of function, as it is often the criterion by which treatment successes are measured. This functionality is influenced by physical as well as psychosocial factors.

Because patients with arthritis will live the remainder of their lives with some degree of their condition, this, indeed, could be one of the most common chronic painful conditions faced in primary care practices today and in the future. Although they are quite different conditions, treatment strategies of OA and RA are similar. These strategies include those listed in Tables 5.10 and 5.11.

■ Table 5.9
Quick Comparison of Osteoarthritis vs. Rheumatoid Arthritis

Osteoarthritis	Rheumatoid Arthritis
Usually occurs in patients 60 years or older	Highest incidence between ages 20 and 50
Asymmetric joint involvement	Symmetric joint involvement
■ Distal and proximal interphalangeal joints	■ Small and large joints
■ Lumbar and cervical spine	Large joint effusion
■ Weight-bearing joints	Inflammatory
Small joint effusion	Stiffness lasts hours to full day
Not inflammatory	Laboratory tests useful
Morning stiffness lasts 20–30 mins	■ Elevated erythrocyte sedimentation rate
Laboratory tests not useful	■ Elevated C-reactive protein
Radiographic evidence	■ Anemia of chronic disease
■ Joint space narrowing of large, weight-bearing joints	■ Rheumatoid factor present in 90% of patients
■ Increased subchondral bony sclerosis	Rheumatoid factor present in 90% of patients
	Radiographic evidence
	■ Variable

■ Table 5.10
Treatment of Arthritis Pain

1. **Patient education**
   a. Weight reduction
   b. Physical exercise
   c. Cognitive-behavioral therapy
   d. Self-help techniques
   e. Good nutritional habits   *(continued)*

■ **Table 5.10**
Treatment of Arthritis Pain *(continued)*

2. **Assistive devices**

   a. Cane

   b. Crutches

   c. Walker

3. It is clear that **altering the progression of disease** in rheumatoid arthritis (RA) has importance in controlling pain. In RA, these drugs are often the first line of therapy. Disease-modifying medications commonly used to achieve this goal include the following:

   a. Methotrexate

   b. Leflunomide

   c. Tumor necrosis factor (TNF-a inhibitors)

   d. Sulfasalazine

4. **Topical agents** may be beneficial in helping to abate arthritis-related pain.

   a. Capsaicin

   b. Lidocaine patch 5%

   c. Diclofenac epolamine topical patch

5. Hyaluronic acid **viscosupplementation** may be useful in treating osteoarthritis (OA) and is Food and Drug Administration–approved for OA of the knee.

6. **Analgesics**

   a. Acetaminophen (in the absence of signs of inflammation)

   b. Nonsteroidal anti-inflammatory drugs

      i. Nonspecific nonsteroidal anti-inflammatory drugs (Consider coadministration of proton pump inhibitor for gastric protection).

      ii. Cyclooxygenase-2–selective nonsteroidal anti-inflammatory drugs (only in appropriate patients)

   c. Intra-articular injection of glucocorticoids in patients with OA with significant inflammation

(continued)

■ **Table 5.10**
  Treatment of Arthritis Pain *(continued)*

---

  d. Systemic glucocorticoids should be avoided in treatment
     of OA, but may be useful in low doses and short-term use
     in treatment of RA.

  i. Should be combined with osteoporosis prophylaxis:

   • Bisphosphonates

   • Calcium supplementation

   • Vitamin D supplementation

7. **Opioids** should be used in patients with OA or RA when other
   medications or nonpharmacologic approaches provide
   inadequate pain relief and affect the patient's quality of life.
   These include but are not limited to the following:

   a. Morphine

   b. Oxycodone

   c. Oxymorphone

   d. Hydrocodone

8. **Tramadol**, like opioids, may be effective in treating pain in OA
   and RA that has been refractory to other treatments.

   Opioids and tramadol may be used in combination with other
   medications and approaches to minimize the dosage of opioid
   required, and therefore minimize adverse effects of these drugs.

■ **Table 5.11**
 Surgical Intervention

Procedures	Reasons for Surgery
Procedures such as synovectomy, arthroscopic debridement, and joint replacement surgery often have improved success rates before the development of tendon rupture, contracture, or advanced joint disease. Commonly, the decision to treat with surgical intervention is made on an individual basis with consideration of the following factors.	Pain
	Function
	Deformity
	Stiffness
	Medical risk factors
	Patient goals and preferences
	Prior treatments and successes
	Radiographic evidence
	Age
	Patient quality of life

Gout

Gout is one of the most painful forms of arthritis. Gout typically is an example of an acutely painful arthritic condition, as compared to OA and RA. Gout accounts for approximately 5% of all cases of arthritis. In the United States, it occurs in approximately 840 out of every 100,000 people. Gout is nine times more common in men than women. Gout often affects men in their 40s and 50s, although gout attacks can occur after puberty, which sees an increase in uric acid levels. Gout attacks are more common in women after the menopause.

Gout is thought to occur from buildup of uric acid in the body, resulting in the following:

■ Sharp uric acid crystal deposits in the joints, typically the big toe

■ Tophi, deposits of uric acid under the skin, appearing as hard lumps

■ Uric acid renal calculi

Although the first attack of gout often occurs in the big toe, it can also occur in other locations, such as in the following:

- Ankles
- Elbows
- Fingers
- Heels
- Instep
- Knees
- Wrist

Commonly, gouty "attacks" can be brought on by stress, alcohol consumption, an acute illness, or even medications. The attacks can last from 3 to 10 days and may be separated from each other by months or even years. Presentation of a gouty attack is usually characteristic, with patients presenting with the following symptoms:

- *Exquisite tenderness* and pain in the big toe
- Often awaking the patient from sleep at the time of the attack
- Redness
- Swelling
- Warmth of the affected area
- Stiffness

In addition to signs and symptoms, the clinician can test to confirm or exclude the diagnosis of gout:

- History of present illness
  - Sudden onset of 1 day of arthritis-like symptoms with redness and swelling
  - Presence in one single joint
- Determination of serum uric acid level
- Examination of joint aspirate for presence of uric acid crystals

■ **Table 5.12**
Treatment of Gout Pain

1. Traditionally, treatment for acute gout has consisted of **colchicine**, which can be effective if given early in the attack (best if used in the first 12 hours of acute attack).

2. **Nonsteroidal anti-inflammatory drugs** can decrease inflammation as well as pain in joints and other tissues. Nonsteroidal anti-inflammatory drugs have become the treatment choice for most acute attacks of gout.

3. **Corticosteroids** are important options in patients who cannot take nonsteroidal anti-inflammatory drugs or colchicine. Given orally or by injection directly into the joint or intramuscularly, they can be very effective in treating gout attacks.

4. **Resting the affected joint** and applying cold compresses to the area also may help alleviate pain.

Neuropathic Pain

Until recently, the mechanisms of neuropathic pain have been unknown. It is currently thought to be due to injury to or dysfunction of the nervous system. There are likely multiple mechanisms of neuropathic pain.[26] Possibilities include the following:

■ Genetic predisposition to develop pain after nerve injury

■ Alteration of the input from peripheral nerves to the dorsal horn of the spinal cord

■ Aberrant growth of sympathetic fibers

■ Peripheral or central sensitization

■ An abnormal inflammatory response. Peripheral nerves, the spinal cord, and the brain react to the environment and change structure and function, emphasizing the plasticity of the nervous system.

Some common causes of neuropathic pain include the following:

■ Alcoholism

■ Amputation

■ Back, leg, and hip problems

- Cancer chemotherapy

- Diabetes

- Facial nerve problems

- Human immunodeficiency virus infection or acquired immunodeficiency syndrome

- Multiple sclerosis

- Shingles [postherpetic neuralgia (PHN)]

- Spine surgery

Assessment of the patient with neuropathic pain involves the standard assessment for pain discussed in Chapter IV. The sensory qualities of neuropathic pain can also be assessed by specific self-report paper and pencil measures. Two instruments that are commonly used are the McGill Pain Questionnaire,[27] an instrument with a long history of research, and the newer, Neuropathic Pain Scale.[28] The Neuropathic Pain Scale is a reliable and valid measure of self-reported pain intensity, especially designed with attention to common aspects of neuropathic pain. A difference between the McGill Pain Questionnaire and the Neuropathic Pain Scale is the manner in which they are scored; the McGill Pain Questionnaire results in a composite score of sensory items and the Neuropathic Pain Scale results in 10 separate scores.

A focused neurologic examination should determine the presence of the following[26]:

- **Allodynia** (the sensation of pain after a stimulus that does not normally evoke pain; allodynia may be experienced by air blowing over the affected area, or light touch, such as the sensation of sheets or clothing)

  - Testing for the presence of dynamic allodynia is accomplished by lightly rubbing the area (e.g., with fingertip or a cotton swab)

  - Static allodynia is found by applying perpendicular pressure (e.g., with a pencil eraser or a cotton swab)

  - Thermal allodynia by applying warm or cold stimuli (e.g., with a test tube or tuning fork)

- **Hyperalgesia** (abnormally increased pain reactions elicited by stimuli that would normally not be painful)
  - Single and multiple pinpricks can be used to test for hyperalgesia
- **Myofascial pain**
  - Tightening muscles, ligaments, and tendons
- **Motor deficiencies**
  - Weakness
  - Ataxia
  - Decreased endurance

Laboratory tests in neuropathic pain, such as neuroradiologic tests and electrophysiologic studies, can sometimes be helpful in establishing the diagnosis but are not helpful in determining the presence or severity of pain.

Neuropathic pain can occur in many syndromes, including diabetic peripheral neuropathy (DPN), PHN, polyneuropathy, central pain syndromes (e.g., poststroke pain, phantom pain), and complex regional pain syndrome (CRPS) (types I and II). Some neuropathic pain states are associated with cancer and include those induced by chemotherapy, impingement of tumor on nerves, radiation, and postsurgical neuropathic pain syndromes (e.g., postmastectomy pain).[25] Painful polyneuropathies are often described as "burning and shooting" with "tingling and pins and needles." They generally occur in a stocking-and-glove distribution.

Treatment algorithms for neuropathic pain based on efficacy, tolerability, safety, and the results of published controlled clinical trials have been suggested by Galer and Dworkin[26] and generally include the following:

- Topical analgesics
- Tricyclic antidepressants
- Anticonvulsants
- Opioids
- Other medications (e.g., tizanidine, tramadol) and selected invasive interventions

Diabetic Peripheral Neuropathy

DPN is an often undiagnosed and tragic complication of diabetes. DPN is thought to occur as a result of microvascular insufficiency, a common complication of diabetes. Twenty-five to fifty percent of diabetic patients develop DPN in their lifetime.[29] Although it occurs so commonly, a recent survey by the American Diabetes Association indicated that for most of the respondents who experienced pain, 75% had not been diagnosed. Additionally, in 2005, 56% of symptomatic respondents were not even familiar with the term "diabetic neuropathy."[30]

DPN can have several deleterious effects on patients, not unlike other chronic painful conditions, including the following:

- Depression
- Anxiety
- Insomnia
- Decreased quality of life
  - Inability to perform activities of daily living
  - Increased disability
  - Inability to perceive dangerous conditions
    - Heat
    - Cold
    - Tissue damage

The most common form of DPN is distal symmetrical polyneuropathy of the lower extremities, manifesting itself with pain having the following qualities:

- Shooting
- Burning
- Stabbing pain in the feet or lower legs

A position statement in 2006 by the American Diabetes Association recommends screening of patients for DPN at the time of diagnosis of type 2 diabetes and 5 years after diagnosis of type 1 diabetes.[31] Screening for DPN includes examination of ankle reflexes and sensory

■ **Table 5.13**
Treatment of Diabetic Peripheral Neuropathy

Treatment of diabetic peripheral neuropathy (DPN) pain is similar to that of other types of neuropathic pain with some special treatments as well, including the following:

1. **Glycemic control** (paramount importance in DPN)

2. **Antidepressants**

   a. **Tricyclics**, such as amitriptyline, nortriptyline, desipramine, doxepin, imipramine, maprotine, and clomipramine

   b. **Selective serotonin reuptake inhibitors**, such as fluoxetine, paroxitene, sertraline, citalopram, and fluvoxamine

   c. Selective norepinephrine and serotonin reuptake inhibitors, such as venlafaxine

   d. Others, such as bupropion, trazodone, nefazodone, and mirtazapine

3. **Anticonvulsants**

   a. **Gabapentin** is often considered to be the first-line oral agent for the treatment of neuropathic pain

   b. **Pregabalin** (recent U.S. Food and Drug Administration approval for treatment of DPN) gives presumed pain-relief at the alpha 2-delta subunit of the presynaptic calcium channel

   c. Others include phenytoin, carbamazepine, topiramate, and valproic acid

4. **Opioids**

5. **Topical analgesics**

   a. Lidocaine patch 5%

   b. Topical capsaicin

6. **Duloxetine** (recent U.S. Food and Drug Administration approval for treatment of DPN) is presumed to have a pain-relieving effect by 5-hydroxytryptamine and norepinephrine reuptake inhibition

7. **Use of well-fitting and cushioned shoes, or athletic shoes**

function in the feet. Investigation should be performed to inquire about neuropathic symptoms in the feet and lower extremities, as well as physical examination for ulcers, sores, or other forms of tissue damage.

The early recognition and appropriate management of neuropathy in the patient with diabetes are important for a number of reasons:

- Nondiabetic neuropathies may be present in patients with diabetes and may be treatable.

- A number of treatment options exist for symptomatic diabetic neuropathy.

- Up to 50% of DPN may be asymptomatic, and patients are at risk of insensate injury to their feet.

- Autonomic neuropathy may involve every system in the body.
  - Cardiovascular autonomic neuropathy causes substantial morbidity and mortality.

Specific treatment for the underlying nerve damage is currently not available, other than improved glycemic control, which may slow progression but rarely reverses neuronal loss. Effective symptomatic treatments are available for the manifestations of DPN and autonomic neuropathy. Once the diagnosis of DPN is established, special foot care is appropriate for insensate feet to decrease the risk of amputation.[31]

Postherpetic Neuralgia

PHN is a painful condition caused by the varicella zoster virus in a dermatomal distribution (the area governed by a particular sensory nerve) after an attack of herpes zoster, usually manifesting after the vesicles have crusted over and begun to heal. Each year, approximately 1 million individuals in the United States develop shingles, or herpes zoster. Approximately 20% of these shingles patients, or 200,000 individuals, go on to suffer from PHN.

PHN is thought to result after nerve fibers are damaged during a case of herpes zoster. Damaged fibers cannot transmit electrical signals from the skin to the brain as they normally do and these signals may be erratic or even exaggerated, causing chronic, often excruciating pain that may persist or recur for months—or even years—in the area where shingles first occurred. Some research suggests that this condition is three times more frequent in the cancer patient population due to immunocompromise.[32]

Pain and temperature detection systems are hypersensitive to light mechanical stimulation, which causes severe pain even from gentle touch or pressure (allodynia). Allodynia may be related to formation of new connections involving central pain transmission neurons. Other patients with PHN may have severe, spontaneous pain without allodynia, possibly secondary to increased spontaneous activity in deafferented central neurons or reorganization of central connections. An imbalance involving loss of large inhibitory fibers and an intact or increased number of small excitatory fibers has been suggested. This input on an abnormal dorsal horn containing deafferented hypersensitive neurons supports the clinical observation that both central and peripheral areas are involved in the production of pain.

In 2006 the FDA approved a herpes zoster vaccine that is recommended for patients who are over age 60 and who have had varicella. The vaccine has been found to decrease the incidence of postherpetic neuralgia by 50%, and the outbreaks that occur are less severe.[33]

Treatments are primarily pharmacologic, as noted in "Neuropathic Pain." In addition to other modalities for treatment of neuropathic pain, the lidocaine patch 5% is a topical patch approved by the FDA for the treatment of PHN. It is effective and extremely well-tolerated and can be safely used in conjunction with other pharmacotherapies because there is no clinically significant absorption of lidocaine. Antiviral agents (e.g., famciclovir) may also be used, the logic being that an antiviral may shorten the clinical course, prevent complications, prevent the development of latency and/or subsequent recurrences, decrease transmission, and eliminate established latency.

Painful Polyneuropathy

Peripheral neuropathy is an umbrella term for a number of patterns of nerve involvement that include mononeuropathy, mononeuropathy multiplex, plexopathy, radiculopathy, and peripheral polyneuropathy. Polyneuropathy can be recognized by classic stocking-and-glove distribution of sensory and motor findings, which in a subgroup of patients is accompanied by pain. The most common causes of peripheral polyneuropathy are diabetes, alcohol use, vitamin deficiencies, hypothyroidism, toxins including medications, and vasculitis. Cryptogenic polyneuropathy (i.e., unknown diagnosis) is a large category; recent evidence suggests that many patients with cryptogenic polyneuropathy have impaired glucose tolerance.

Diabetes may cause a number of different types of neuropathy; peripheral polyneuropathy is the most common, but other types include the following:

- Diabetic amyotrophy

- Thoracic radiculopathy

- Autonomic neuropathy

- Third cranial neuropathy

The most important goal in a patient presenting with a peripheral neuropathy is to make the diagnosis because many of the neuropathies can be resolved or stabilized with primary treatment. It is of critical importance to make a diagnosis because disorders that require prompt recognition sometimes masquerade as a "benign" peripheral polyneuropathy. Once the diagnosis is established, or concurrently with diagnostic efforts, the pain must be managed.

Management is basically pharmacologic, analogous to the approach to neuropathic pain in general. Because the area of pain is often widespread in patients with peripheral polyneuropathy, the topical agents may be less practical than in focal neuropathies; in fact, they are increasingly used and may be helpful for focal neuropathies. The oral medication approach is analogous to other types of neuropathic pain.

Complex Regional Pain Syndrome

CRPS (*type I*), formerly referred to as *reflex sympathetic dystrophy*, is a painful condition that usually develops after minor trauma, such as a sprain, strain, or contusion. CRPS type I may also follow bony fracture, surgery, or relatively benign soft tissue injury. CRPS (*type II*), formerly referred to as *causalgia*, develops after injury to a large nerve (e.g., a gunshot wound to nerve or plexus). CRPS most commonly occurs near or at the site of injury (e.g., in one hand or foot) but can be found in other body parts and may spread from the original site. The spread of pain in CRPS can be related to myofascial dysfunction in proximal muscles or may represent a centralization of the pain process, including a somatoform process.

CRPS is usually described by patients presenting with the following complaints:

- Pain
  - Burning
  - Deep aching
  - Lancinating
- Allodynia
- Edema
- Skin color changes (e.g., mottled, red, blotchy)
- Skin temperature changes (hot or cold compared with the contralateral side of the body)
- Motor weakness
- Sweating (increased or decreased compared to the contralateral side)
- Brittle nails
- Other nonspecific skin changes (e.g., shiny or extremely dry)
- Various movement disorders affecting the involved limb

The allodynia that patients present with is a characteristic feature that often interferes with the patient's ability to tolerate clothing, air conditioning, or any type of touch in the affected area. CRPS is a clinical diagnosis, and the International Association for the Study of Pain has provided diagnostic guidelines.[34]

Treatment for CRPS can be quite challenging, and usually involves a variety of modalities, including diagnostic and therapeutic nerve blocks, medications, and physiotherapy. Pharmacologic interventions include the following:

- Lidocaine patch 5%
- Gabapentin or pregabalin
- Intravenous lidocaine
- Mexiletine
- Opioids
- Tricyclic antidepressants
- Tizanidine

Spinal cord stimulation has been efficacious for selected individuals but is only recommended when other more conservative treatments have failed. Finally, patients with true cases of CRPS almost always require psychological treatments designed to increase their pain-coping skills, decrease negative affect (e.g., depression and anxiety), and provide support through a course of rehabilitation that is often difficult.

Pain Syndromes from Peripheral Nerve Injury

Pain syndromes as a result of direct peripheral nerve injury include the following:

- Postthoracotomy pain
  - Affects the intercostal nerves and is often described as an "aching" sensation in the distribution of the incision
- Postmastectomy pain
- Postnephrectomy pain
  - Associated with nerves in the superficial flank and is described as numbness, fullness, or heaviness in the flank

- Various pain syndromes after amputation
  - The most common types of pain after amputation are phantom pain and stump pain, which are distinguished by the location of the pain being either in the "phantom" of the amputated limb or in its stump, respectively.
  - May be manifested by the following:
    - Burning dysesthesia
    - Cramping
    - Feelings of distorted posturing of the nonexistent limb

The treatment of focal neuropathic pain syndromes in general follows the World Health Organization (WHO) algorithm with a focus on neuropathic pain syndromes. Although not well-studied, interventional procedures, such as scar injections with steroids or neurolytic agents (e.g., phenol or alcohol), neurolytic blocks (e.g., subarachnoid alcohol), or epidural or intrathecal analgesia, can be quite useful.

Plexopathy

Plexopathy is a major cause of pain in cancer patients. It is produced by tumor invasion or compression of the cervical, brachial, or lumbosacral plexuses or as a consequence of radiation therapy. Pain is more common in plexopathy due to tumor invasion than in radiation plexopathy, wherein general neurological deficits are more prominent. It should be noted that pain may precede overt neurologic signs in plexopathies. Distinguishing plexopathy due to tumor from plexopathy due to radiation may be difficult; in general, the distinction is based on the clinical picture, imaging studies, and electrophysiologic studies.

Pain related to the cervical plexus is usually experienced in the face or head and is described as lancinating, burning, or aching. Swallowing or head movement can intensify the pain. It is important to distinguish cervical plexopathy from epidural compression, which can be done through magnetic resonance imaging or computed tomographic imaging.

Brachial plexopathy is associated with cancers of the lung or breast, with most cases associated with upper lobe lung cancer.[35] Pain in the lower plexus usually involves pain in the shoulder that extends to the arm and fourth and fifth digits. Pain in the upper plexus, which occurs less frequently, begins in the shoulder, lateral arm, index finger, and thumb. Brachial plexopathy is usually diagnosed by computed tomographic imaging or magnetic resonance imaging. Patients with lumbosacral plexopathy usually experience pain in the pelvis, buttock, and legs. Similar to cervical and brachial plexuses, lumbosacral plexopathy can be assessed by magnetic resonance imaging or computed tomographic imaging.

Treatment of the plexopathies, again, focuses on diagnosis, primary treatment when available, and analgesic treatment, more or less in parallel. Analgesic treatment proceeds according to the WHO ladder, described in "World Health Organization Analgesic Ladder for Cancer Pain," with a focus on neuropathic pain medications. Interventional treatments can be quite effective in plexopathy pain, which is often intractable to medical management. In particular, subarachnoid alcohol neurolysis, which is in experienced hands a relatively simple and safe outpatient procedure, relieves pain reliably for a few months in most patients. Patients may also do well with prolonged epidural or intrathecal analgesic modalities, but these procedures are in general much more difficult than the neurolytic procedures under an experienced operator.

Peripheral Polyneuropathies

Peripheral polyneuropathies can be recognized by the classic stocking-and-glove distribution of symptoms and signs, as discussed previously in the case of the noncancer patient. Peripheral polyneuropathies can be caused by chemotherapy (e.g., vinca alkaloids, paclitaxel, cisplatin, docetaxel, and vinorelbine tartrate), nutritional deficiencies, metabolic problems, alcohol consumption, and other causes. Of course, identification and treatment, when possible, of the underlying cause of the neuropathy are the most important initial steps.

Symptomatic treatment of these syndromes involves the cascade of medical treatments for neuropathic pain described on page 90, which may lead to implantable analgesic infusion pumps or spinal cord stimulators.

Central Pain Syndrome

Central pain syndrome is a neurologic condition caused by damage to or dysfunction of the central nervous system. This syndrome can be caused by the following:

- Cerebrovascular accident

- Brain or spinal cord trauma

- Epilepsy

- Multiple sclerosis

- Parkinson's disease

- Tumor-based causes (e.g., direct pressure, tissue infiltration)

The character of the pain associated with this syndrome varies widely and may affect a large portion of the body or may be more restricted to specific areas, such as hands or feet. The extent of pain is usually related to the cause of the central nervous system injury or damage.[36]

Patients present with the following signs and symptoms and one of the above conditions:

- Pain that is typically constant
  - Moderate to severe in intensity
  - Worsened by touch, movement, emotions, and temperature changes, usually cold temperatures
  - One or more types of pain sensations, the most prominent being burning
    - Mingled with the burning may be sensations of the following:
      - "Pins and needles"
      - Pressing
      - Lacerating or aching pain
      - Brief, intolerable bursts of sharp pain, similar to dental nerve pain

■ Individuals may have numbness in the areas affected by the pain

Central pain syndrome often begins shortly after the causative injury or damage, but may be delayed by months or even years, especially if it is related to post-cerebrovascular accident pain. Treatment includes conventional agents used in managing neuropathic pain, including tricyclics, anticonvulsants, and stress reduction.

Fibromyalgia

Although fibromyalgia (often referred to as *Fibromyalgia Syndrome* or FMS) has been recognized as a clinical condition since 1987, controversy surrounding its acceptance as a bona fide diagnosis continues. Dr. Frederick Wolfe, the lead author of the original paper that described the diagnostic guidelines for fibromyalgia,[37] was recently quoted as having had second thoughts as to whether it is a unique condition, or actually a constellation of conditions, with depression playing a major role. Despite this controversy, the American College of Rheumatology (ACR), readily recognizes fibromyalgia as a diagnosable *syndrome*, and the European League Against Rheumatism (EULAR), recently published a set of management guidelines for fibromyalgia syndrome in the *Annals of the Rheumatic Diseases*.[38] EULAR plans to update the guidelines every 5 years, and incorporate findings from good quality clinical trials that will add to currently available evidence.

Fibromyalgia was formerly known as *fibrositis*, and is considered to be one of the rheumatic diseases, although its etiology is currently unknown. Researchers have found elevated levels of a nerve chemical signal, called substance P, and nerve growth factor in the spinal fluid of fibromyalgia patients. Serotonin is also relatively low in patients with fibromyalgia. Studies of pain in fibromyalgia have suggested that the central nervous system may be somehow super-sensitized. The painful muscle tissue involved is not accompanied by tissue inflammation. Therefore, despite potentially disabling body pain, patients with fibromyalgia do not develop body damage or deformity.

The 1990 ACR criteria for classification of fibromyalgia included:

1. **History of widespread pain**, defined as widespread when all of the following are present: pain in the left side of the body,

pain in the right side of the body, pain above the waist, and pain below the waist. In addition, axial skeletal pain (cervical spine or anterior chest or thoracic spine or low back) must be present. In this definition, shoulder and buttock pain is considered as pain for each involved side. "Low back" pain is considered lower segment pain. The widespread pain must be present for 3 months duration or longer.

2. **Pain in 11 of 18 specific tender point sites** on digital palpation. Tender points are located on either side of the neck, chest, upper back, lower back, spine, buttocks, knee caps, or the inside of either arm where it bends at the elbow.

For classification purposes, patients will be said to have fibromyalgia if both criteria are satisfied.

This condition is thought to affect 2–7% of the general population, and is characterized by pain, stiffness, and tenderness of the muscles, tendons, and joints. This very challenging condition is more common in women, and tends to develop during early and middle adulthood or during a woman's childbearing years. Those who have another rheumatic disease such as lupus, rheumatoid arthritis, or ankylosing spondylitis, also are at a higher risk for developing fibromyalgia.

The diagnosis of fibromyalgia may be made based on the ACR criteria, or based on the presence of the characteristic syndrome, or both, and the presence of a second clinical disorder does not exclude the diagnosis of fibromyalgia. Patients typically present with the following complaints:

- Chronic widespread muscular pain (3 months duration or longer)
- Chronic fatigue
- Widespread tenderness (hyperalgesia)

Many people with fibromyalgia also experience additional symptoms, such as the following:

- Morning stiffness
- Headaches

- Irritable bowel syndrome
- Irritable bladder
- Cognitive and memory problems (often called "fibro fog")
- Symptoms of temporo-mandibular joint disorder
- Pelvic pain

A number of clinicians are often concerned that patients with fibromyalgia syndrome suffer from comorbid psychological conditions, such as depression as well. This is likely due to the large number of varying complaints from these patients, and the high incidence of depression in these patients. The likelihood is that these patients are suffering from a high incidence of anxiety and depression as a result of their widespread chronic pain. The EULAR Guidelines address some of these concerns in their recommendations for management of patients with FMS, which include:

- Comprehensive evaluation of pain, function, and psychosocial context is needed to understand FMS completely, because it is a complex, heterogeneous condition involving abnormal pain processing and other secondary features

- Optimal treatment of FMS mandates a multidisciplinary approach, which should include a combination of nonpharmacologic and pharmacologic interventions. After discussion with the patient, treatment modalities should be specifically tailored based on pain intensity, function, and associated features such as depression, fatigue, and sleep disturbance

- Cognitive behavioral therapy, relaxation, rehabilitation, physiotherapy, psychological support, and other modalities may be indicated for certain patients

Treatment is with conventional therapies and usually includes an antidepressant. Pregabalin, an anticonvulsant used for the treatment of neuropathic pain, such as diabetic peripheral neuropathy, and post-herpetic neuralgia, has recently been approved by the Food and Drug Administration for treatment of pain and improving impairment of daily function related to FMS, as it has shown to be effective in treating some patients with fibromyalgia. Additionally, therapeutic regimens include exercise programs, analgesics, and behavioral therapy. The goals of treatment for fibromyalgia are to control pain and improve function.

Myofascial Pain

Myofascial pain is defined as a syndrome consisting of pain in a muscle, which is usually in spasm, and contains taut bands and/or trigger points, palpation of which reproduces the patient's pain, often with a radiating component.[39]

Associated symptoms may include heaviness, "numbness" without neurologic signs, swelling, or decreased range of motion. Trigger points are defined as localized palpable mass within a muscle, palpation of which reproduces the patient's pain, including the radiating component.[40] Myofascial pain is a regional disorder, as opposed to fibromyalgia, which by definition is a widespread disorder. Another distinction is that fibromyalgia is characterized by tender points (which are tender, but nothing is palpable), as opposed to the trigger points of myofascial pain. Myofascial pain is a clinical diagnosis. A variety of stress-producing stimuli have been postulated in the etiology and maintenance of myofascial pain, including physical stress (e.g., fatigue), tissue injury (major or microtrauma), physiologic state (e.g., hormonal balance, nutritional status), personality, and genetic factors.[41]

Myofascial syndromes are treated by physical interventions, such as stretching, strengthening, postural reeducation, other forms of physical therapy, and vapocoolant sprays. Cases that do not respond to conservative therapy can be successfully treated with trigger point injections of a local anesthetic, low-dose steroid, or saline. Recent reports have suggested the efficacy of botulinum toxin in the treatment of refractory cases.[42] Complaints of myofascial pain, especially in the setting of headache, LBP, and CRPS type I, are common and can result from disuse of muscles secondary to pain.

Chronic Abdominal Pain

Abdominal pain can be the result of a variety of causes that individually are beyond the scope of this manual. Some examples of causes of abdominal pain are chronic intestinal obstructive processes, which occur frequently in the setting of abdominal and pelvic cancers. Other causes include visceral tumors (primary or metastatic), venous thrombosis, omental metastases, volvulus of the small intestine, and occlusion of blood flow to visceral organs. Because the issue of decreased bowel motility is quite important in this group of patients, adjunctive treatments and medications, in addition to opioids to spare the adverse effects, are often used. Adjunctive treatments include subcutaneous infusion of octreotide, antispasmodic agents, and antiemetics. Interventional treatments include neurolytic procedures (e.g., celiac or hypogastric plexus block, which are contraindicated in the presence of bowel obstruction) and spinal analgesic infusions.

Cancer Pain

Although research indicates that the majority of patients with cancer experience some form of pain, pain associated with cancer is frequently left undertreated. Notably, untreated cancer pain is a major risk factor for suicide. Even though cancer pain cannot usually be entirely relieved, several treatment strategies exist to help to alleviate much of the pain and therefore improve the patient's quality of life.

Lack of effective treatment is most often due to inadequate screening and assessment. The goals of screening are twofold:

1. To screen patients routinely to determine the presence and extent of pain

2. To make a diagnosis in patients who have pain

Various barriers in the clinician-patient interaction frequently prevent the recognition of pain when it is present, without which diagnosis and treatment can never take place. The purpose of diagnosis is, as is the case with any pain syndrome, to determine whether a primary treatment exists for the underlying cause of the pain. For example, many patients with cancer develop new sources of pain that are due to treatable infections.[43]

The patient's description of the pain leading to its categorization as *somatic*, *visceral*, or *neuropathic*, is a critical guide to treatment. In cancer pain, *somatic pain* can result from tumor invasion (by direct growth or metastasis) of the bone and muscle. *Visceral pain* commonly occurs in the setting of malignancies involving internal organ systems, such as the pancreas, uterus, or liver. *Neuropathic pain* can be caused by malignant invasion and subsequent damage or disruption of peripheral nerves, plexuses, nerve root, spinal cord, or brain. Frequently, the type of cancer pain is of mixed origin. (For further definitions of the types of pain, refer to Chapter I in the manual or the glossary.) Although opioids are helpful in many types of cancer pain, they are not necessarily the most appropriate first-line treatment for certain types of pain (e.g., mild bone pain), and in some cases are minimally effective.

A psychosocial assessment is also important. Consider the effect of the cancer diagnosis on the patient, the patient's coping responses, the patient's knowledge of pain management and concerns about using controlled substances, the economic effect of pain, and changes in mood.

The diagnostic evaluation of the cause of the pain may require blood tests, radiologic studies, or neurophysiologic testing. Finally, assessment of pain at regular intervals should be ongoing.[35]

Two common cancer pain problems include the following:

- **Peri-procedural pain**
  - Generally as a result of biopsy or removal of the cancerous tissue or organ
  - Treatment resembles that of any other acute source of peri-procedural pain

- **Bony metastasis**
  - The most common cause of pain in cancer patients and is often associated with cancers of the lung, prostate, and breast. The most common areas in which they form are in the vertebrae, pelvis, femur, and skull. In many cases, patients have multiple areas of bone metastases. and therefore have multiple areas of pain. Such pain is usually described as dull and aching.

- A diagnosis of bony metastasis is confirmed through radiographic testing.
- Treatment consists of the following:
  - Primary treatment of the cancer
  - Radiation therapy is often widely used for metastatic bone pain and is highly effective and generally well-tolerated.
  - Pharmacologic management
    - Nonsteroidal anti-inflammatory drugs may be more effective than opioids, especially for movement-associated pain.
    - Many clinicians prescribed selective COX-2 inhibitors, but now recognize risks associated with these drugs. This drug class still represents a viable option in carefully selected patients.
    - Opioids and other pharmacologic treatments should be added if needed, as discussed in the "Pharmacologic Options for the Management of Pain" section in Chapter VI.
    - Patients who do not respond adequately to medical management should be referred for pain management consultation because they may respond well to intrathecal analgesia or other interventional procedures.

A growing concern in oncology is a new kind of cancer patient, one who has the long-term pain issues of a cancer survivor. This kind of chronic pain requires a treatment approach that is much more like that of noncancer chronic pain. One of the common reasons for chronic pain in cancer survivors is chemotherapy induced plexitis and postsurgical pain syndromes. Unfortunately, a significant percentage of patients who undergo chemotherapy and other treatment modalities for cancer will experience this long-term pain problem.

Treatment of Cancer Pain

The treatment of cancer pain involves both pharmacologic and nonpharmacologic interventions. In terms of pharmacologic treatment, the

WHO has developed an effective guideline for titration of analgesic therapy for cancer pain, which has become known as the *analgesic ladder*.[35]

World Health Organization Analgesic Ladder for Cancer Pain. The WHO in 1990 and 1996 issued guidelines that involve the treatment of cancer pain. The guidelines are presented in a ladder formation and are referred to as the "analgesic ladder." The steps of the WHO ladder are described in Figure 3 and Table 5.14.

■ **Figure 3**
WHO Analgesic Ladder for Cancer Pain

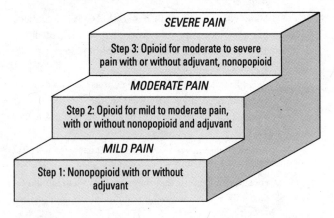

SEVERE PAIN

Step 3: Opioid for moderate to severe pain with or without adjuvant, nonopopioid

MODERATE PAIN

Step 2: Opioid for mild to moderate pain, with or without nonopopioid and adjuvant

MILD PAIN

Step 1: Nonopopioid with or without adjuvant

■ **Table 5.14**
World Health Organization Analgesic Ladder for Cancer Pain

Step 1

The first step involves treatment of mild to moderate pain with acetaminophen, aspirin, or another nonsteroidal anti-inflammatory drug. Medications should be administered as needed or round-the-clock and should be titrated upward when necessary. Adjuvant analgesics, or medications that are not generally used for pain (but can have an enhancing effect on other analgesics), may also be used. *(continued)*

■ **Table 5.14**
World Health Organization Analgesic Ladder
for Cancer Pain *(continued)*

Step 2

The second step involves adding an opioid for pain that persists beyond treatment in step 1. An opioid, often codeine or oxycodone, is added to the regimen at this step (the nonsteroidal anti-inflammatory drug or acetaminophen should be retained).

Step 3

The third step involves treatment with an opioid on a round-the-clock basis for persistent pain. Morphine is generally the agent of choice. Short-acting opioids are often prescribed as needed for pain as a supplement to a "background dose" of long-acting opioids. This type of dosing is called "rescue" or "breakthrough" and is given for exacerbations of pain that occur beyond the constant, background pain. Whenever possible, the same type of opioid should be given for background and breakthrough treatment.

---

1. **The World Health Organization (WHO) approach to pharmacologic treatment contains five major concepts:**

   a. By the mouth

   b. By the clock

   c. By the ladder

   d. For the individual

   e. With careful documentation

2. In treating patients with cancer, the medication regimen should be individualized. A simple regimen should be developed, and medication should be taken orally unless the patient is unable (e.g., trouble swallowing, obtundation).

3. **Nonsteroidal anti-inflammatory drugs** and/or acetaminophen should be prescribed for mild to moderate pain (**step 1 of the WHO ladder**).

4. With persistent pain or when pain increases, **opioids** should be administered in addition to the nonsteroidal anti-inflammatory drugs. The WHO guidelines initially recommended using **"weak" opioids** for initial treatment—for example, codeine, oxycodone, propoxyphene, hydrocodone, and tramadol (**step 2 of the WHO ladder**).

5. When pain is more severe at the outset or in the case of failure of "weak" opioids, the guidelines recommended using **"strong" opioids**—for example, morphine, hydromorphone, methadone, levorphanol, fentanyl, oxymorphone, and meperidine (**step 3 of the WHO ladder**).

6. These days, the concepts of "strong" and "weak" opioids have been discredited for most clinical situations, and most clinicians would advocate a modified approach to the WHO ladder:

   a. **Start with nonsteroidal anti-inflammatory drugs (cyclooxygenase-2 inhibitors might be a choice in selected patients).**

   b. **Add a short-acting opioid on an as-needed basis if needed.**

   c. **Then add a long-acting opioid on a round-the-clock basis if needed.**

   d. **Adjuvant medications should be added whenever indicated.**

7. Medications should be administered on a regular basis, plus on an as-needed basis, which helps build a constant level of the medication in the body, but also addresses exacerbations of pain, which may be provoked by increased activity during treatment.

8. It is worth emphasizing that patients should enter the rung of the ladder appropriate for their presentation. For example, patients presenting with severe and continuous pain should usually be treated with "strong" opioids at the beginning, which may be most effectively administered intravenously in the acute setting. Patients can then be transitioned, once pain is under control,

to a regimen consisting of a nonsteroidal anti-inflammatory drug, a sustained-release opioid, plus a short-acting opioid for breakthrough pain.

9. Long-term opioid use may be associated with tolerance and physical dependence; however, neither tolerance nor physical dependence generally reflects aberrant (drug-abusing) behavior. Finally, because of the potential for serious side effects, patients should be monitored and evaluated regularly.

End-of-Life Considerations

There is growing recognition of the importance of caring for patients (and their families) with progressive disease that is no longer curable, through the integrated efforts of hospice and palliative care programs. This is not just a concern for patients with cancer pain, but for many other painful conditions as well. Further discussion of this topic is in Chapter VII, Pain Management in Special Patient Populations, under Hospice and Palliative Care.

REFERENCES

1. Apfelbaum JL, Chen C, Mehta SS, Gan TJ. Postoperative pain experience: results from a national survey suggest postoperative pain continues to be undermanaged. *Anesth Analg*. 2003 Aug;97(2):534–540.

2. Mitra S, Sinatra RS. Perioperative management of acute pain in the opioid-dependent patient. *Anesthesiology*. 2004 Jul;101(1):212–227.

3. de Leon-Casasola O, Yarussi A. Pathophysiology of opioid tolerance and clinical approach to the opioid-tolerant patient. *Curr Rev Pain*. 2000;4(3):203–205.

4. O'Brien C. Drug addiction and drug abuse. In Hardman JG, Limbird LE, eds. *Goodman & Gilman's The Pharmacological Basis of Therapeutics*. 10th ed. New York: McGraw-Hill; 2001:621–642.

5. Collett BJ. Chronic opioid therapy for non-cancer pain. *Br J Anaesth*. 2001;87:133–43.

6. Long DM. Chronic back pain. In: Wall PD, Melzack R, eds. *Textbook of Pain*. London: Churchill; 1999:539–558.

7. Roper Public Affairs & Media. *Americans Living with Pain Survey*. Conducted for the American Chronic Pain Association. New York: GFK NOP, 2004.

8. Cooper JK, Kohlmann T. Factors associated with health status of older Americans. *Age Ageing*. 2001 Nov;30(6):495–501.

9. Blount BW, Hart G, Ehreth JL. A description of the content of army family practice. *J Am Board Fam Pract*. 1993 Mar–Apr;6(2):143-52.

10. Carey TS, Garrett JM, Jackman AM. Beyond the good prognosis. Examination of an inception cohort of patients with chronic low back pain. *Spine (Phila PA 1976)*. 2000 Jan;25(1):115–20.

11. National Institutes of Health, National Institute of Neurological Disorders and Stroke (NINDS). Low back pain fact sheet. NIH pub no 03–5161, July 2003. http://www.ninds.nih.gov/disorders/backpain/detail_backpain.htm. Accessed June 28, 2010.

12. Koes BW, van Tulder MW, Ostelo R, Kim Burton A, Waddell G. Clinical guidelines for the management of low back pain in primary care: an international comparison. *Spine (Phila Pa 1976)*. 2001 Nov 15;26(22):2504–13; discussion 2513–4.

13. Deyo RA, Weinstein JN. Low back pain. *N Engl J Med*. 2001 Feb 1;344(5):363–70.

14. Deyo RA, Mirza SK, Martin BI. Back pain prevalence and visit rates: estimates from U.S. national surveys, 2002. *Spine (Phila Pa 1976)*. 2006 Nov 1;31(23):2724–7.

15. Nadler SF, Steiner DJ, Erasala GN, et al. Continuous low-level heat wrap therapy provides more efficacy than Ibuprofen and acetaminophen for acute low back pain. *Spine (Phila Pa 1976)*. 2002 May 15;27(10):1012–7.

16. Chou R, Qaseem A, Snow V, et al. Diagnosis and treatment of low-back pain: a joint clinical practice guideline from the American College of Physicians and the American Pain Society. *Ann Inter Med*. 2007 Oct 2;147(7):478–91.

17. Headache Classification Subcommittee of the International Headache Society. The International Classification of Headache Disorders. 2nd edition. *Cephalalgia*. 2004;24 Suppl 1:9–160.

18. Saper JR, Silberstein S, Gordon CD, et al. *Handbook of Headache Management: A Practical Guide to Diagnosis and Treatment of Head, Neck, and Facial Pain*. Philadelphia: Lippincott Williams & Wilkins; 1999.

19. Schoenen J, Sandor PS. Headache. In: Wall PD, Melzack R, eds. *Textbook of Pain*. London: Churchill; 1999:761–798.

20. Hootman JM, Bolen J, Helmick CG, Langmaid G. Prevalence of doctor-diagnosed arthritis and arthritis-attributable activity limitation—United States, 2003-2005. *MMWR*. 2006;55(40):1089–1092.

21. Hootman JM, Helmick CG. Projections of U.S. prevalence of arthritis and associated activity limitations. *Arthritis Rheum*. 2006;54(1):266–229.

22. Centers for Disease Control and Prevention (CDC). National and state medical expenditures and lost earnings attributable to arthritis and other rheumatic conditions--United States, 2003. *MMWR Morb Mortal Wkly Rep*. 2007 Jan 12;56(1):4–7.

23. Lawrence RC, Felson DT, Helmick CG, et al. Estimates of the prevalence of arthritis and other rheumatic conditions in the United States. Part II. *Arthritis Rheum*. 2008 Jan;58(1):26–35.

24. Zhang W, Moskowitz RW, Nuki G, et al. OARSI recommendations for the management of hip and knee osteoarthritis, Part II: OARSI evidence-based, expert consensus guidelines. *Osteoarthritis Cartilage*. 2008 Feb;16(2):137–62.

25. Harris ED, Zorab R. *Rheumatoid Arthritis*. Philadelphia, PA: WB Saunders Company; 1997.

26. Galer BS, Dworkin RH. *A Clinical Guide to Neuropathic Pain*. New York: The McGraw-Hill Companies; 2000.

27. Melzack R, Casey KL. Sensory motivational and central control determinants of pain: a new conceptual model. In: Kenshalo DR, ed. *The Skin Senses*. Springfield: Thomas; 1968:423–443.

28. Galer BS, Jensen MP. Development and preliminary validation of a pain measure specific to neuropathic pain: the Neuropathic Pain Scale. *Neurology*. 1997;48:332–338.

29. Dyck PJ, Kratz KM, Karnes JL, et al. The prevalence by staged severity of various types of diabetic neuropathy, retinopathy, and nephropathy in a population-based cohort: the Rochester Diabetic Neuropathy Study. *Neurology*. 1993;43:817–824.

30. American Diabetes Association. American Diabetes Association nationwide telephone survey results. *What you don't know about diabetic neuropathy can hurt you*. 2005.

31. American Diabetes Association. Standards of medical care in diabetes. *Diabetes Care*. 2006 Jan;29 Suppl 1:S4–42.

32. Cherny NI, Portenoy RK. Cancer pain: principles of assessment and syndromes. In: Wall PD, Melzack R, eds. *Textbook of Pain*. London: Churchill; 1999:1017–1064.

33. Centers for Disease Control and Prevention (CDC). Recommendations of the Advisory Committee on Immunization Practices (ACIP): prevention of herpes zoster. *MMWR Morb Mortal Wkly Rep*. 2008 May;57:1–30.

34. Bruehl S, Harden RN, Galer BS, et al. External validation of IASP diagnostic criteria for complex regional pain syndrome and proposed research diagnostic criteria. *Pain*. 1999;81:147–154.

35. Jacox AK, Carr DB, Payne R, et al. Management of Cancer Pain, Clinical Practice Guidelines. No. 9. Rockville, MD: U.S. Department of Health and Human Services, Public Health Service, Agency for Health Care Policy and Research (AHCPR Publication No. 94-0592), 1994.

36. National Institute of Neurological Disorders and Stroke. NINDS Central Pain Syndrome Information Page. http://www.ninds.nih.gov/disorders/central_pain/central_pain.htm. Accessed June 29, 2010.

37. Wolfe F, Smythe HA, Yunus MB, et al. The American College of Rheumatology 1990 criteria for the classification of fibromyalgia: report of the multicenter criteria committee. *Arthritis Rheum*. 1990;33: 160–72.

38. Carville SF, Arendt-Nielsen S, Bliddal H, et al. EULAR evidence-based recommendations for the management of fibromyalgia syndrome. *Ann Rheum Dis*. 2008 Apr;67:536–541.

39. Travell JG, Simons DG. *Myofascial Pain and Dysfunction: The Trigger Point Manual*. Baltimore: Williams; 1992.

40. Fisher AA. Documentation of myofascial trigger points. *Arch Phys Med Rehabil*. 1988;69:286–291.

41. Dommerholt J, Shah JP. Myofascial Pain Syndrome. In: Fishman SM, Ballantyne JC, Rathmell JP, eds. *Bonica's Management of Pain*. 4th ed. Philadelphia: Lippincott Williams & Wilkins; 2009:450-471.

42. Cheshire W, Abashian SW, Mann JD. Botulinum toxin in the treatment of myofascial pain syndrome. *Pain*. 1994;59:65–69.

43. Gonzales GR, Elliott KJ, Portenoy RK, Foley KM. The impact of a comprehensive evaluation in the management of cancer pain. *Pain*. 1991;47:141–144.

VI.

Approaches to the Management of Pain

NONPHARMACOLOGIC OPTIONS FOR THE MANAGEMENT OF PAIN

The biopsychosocial model encompasses biologic, psychological, and social aspects of pain. Nonpharmacologic options for the management of pain can be divided into physical, psychological, and psychosocial dimensions.

Physical Modalities

Therapeutic Exercise

Therapeutic exercise includes the following:

- Range-of-motion exercises
- Stretching
- Strength training
- Cardiovascular conditioning

Range-of-motion exercises can be delivered in a passive, assisted-active, or active manner. Multiple exercise techniques in each of these categories can be used to increase physical functioning. Although exercise is generally limited to range of motion during acute pain,[1] patients with chronic pain should be encouraged to *adopt an exercise program as early as possible*. Exercise mobilizes joints and strengthens muscles, in addition to enhancing balance and coordination. Cardiovascular conditioning is also important for maintenance of long-term health.[2] Facilitating exercise should be considered one of the primary goals of analgesic therapy. Randomized clinical trial evidence is strong that physical or restorative therapy should be used for patients with low back pain and other chronic conditions.[3]

Patients may become discouraged when their pain actually increases due to therapeutic exercise. Many patients terminate their treatment far too early to achieve maximal benefit. Health care providers can take this into consideration by choosing to refer to physical therapists who specialize in effectively treating people with chronic pain and who can encourage and motivate them to persist with an exercise program.

Because the primary goal of treatment for individuals with chronic pain is to restore overall functioning, and injuries or disease often diminish physical capacities, the importance of evaluation and treatment with physical measures cannot be underestimated. Before beginning therapy, the physical therapist evaluates range of motion with an instrument called a *goniometer*. The therapist also determines whether restricted motion results from tight muscles or from tight ligaments and tendons.

There are three types of range of motion exercises that are often used:

- **Active exercise:** Exercising a muscle or joint without help.

- **Active-assistive exercise:** Exercising a muscle or joint with help.

- **Passive exercise:** Exercise for people who cannot actively participate. No effort is required from the patient.

Application of Heat and Cold

Early interventions for acute injuries can be **r**est, **i**ce, **c**ompression, and **e**levation, which can be remembered by the popular acronym **RICE**. These interventions are directed at diminishing swelling and inflammation and are most often effective between 24 and 48 hours after an acute injury.[4]

The application of heat can be made via hot packs, hot water bottles, moist compresses, heating pads, chemical and gel packs, and immersion in water.[5] Cold can also be applied to reduce inflammation via ice packs, towels soaked in cold water, or gel packs.

The use of heat and cold therapies is somewhat controversial for cancer pain because of the possible risk of increasing tumor growth. Superficial heat is not contraindicated in some recent cancer guidelines.[5,6] However, caution should be exercised for application of deep heat, including by short wave, microwave, and ultrasound.[5] Heat is also contraindicated for acute musculoskeletal injuries because it can result in increases in hemorrhage and edema.[7]

Care should always be taken for superficial and deep heat and cold delivery, especially for the following patients:

- Individuals with insensate tissue
- Cognitively impaired individuals
- Patients with peripheral vascular disease
- Patients with a bleeding diathesis
- Individuals with metastatic tumors

Physical Manipulation

For *acute pain*, physical manipulation, such as instruction on repositioning and appropriate ways to rise from bed or a chair, is an important component of therapy. For example, physical manipulation can help postsurgical patients reduce movement related pain, early in the course of the postoperative period.

Short-term immobilization of joints or restriction of movement is often necessary to manage painful joints and facilitate healing. Immobilization of joints at angles that approximate the angle of their optimal functioning (e.g., wrist joints at 30 degrees of dorsiflexion) increase functioning when the immobilization is no longer necessary.[8]

For *chronic pain*, although immobilization can be helpful in the short-term, the benefits are generally outweighed by undesired consequences (e.g., contracture, atrophy, and cardiovascular deconditioning) if used on a long-term basis.[8]

Therapeutic Massage

Massage can be delivered by stroking, kneading, pressing, or rhythmic motions, singly or in combination.[9,10] Massage[11] is also considered to be a complementary medicine **treatment**. From a scientific perspective, although massage has been studied in several randomized clinical trials, most of them have methodological weaknesses.[12]

Therapeutic benefits of massage can include the following:

- A sense of relaxation

- Reduction of muscle tension

- Promotion of circulation

- Improvement in sleep

- Decreased pain[10,13]

- Release of endorphins[11]

Transcutaneous Electrical Stimulation

Transcutaneous electrical nerve stimulation (TENS) is a counter-stimulation technique that is thought to stimulate peripheral nerves directly and alter painful sensations. TENS involves applying low-voltage electrical stimulation to large nerve fibers. Patients report that a "tingling" sensation replaces painful sensations. TENS has been shown to provide effective pain relief in some forms of acute pain conditions, including postoperative pain, oral-facial pain, and pain associated with childbearing.[14] However, the results of research for TENS in chronic pain are mixed,[15] and more rigorous, large multi-center randomized clinical trials are needed.[16]

Some manufacturers of electrical TENS units indicate that TENS over a cancer site is contraindicated. "Cancer guidelines state that TENS may be beneficial for patients with mild cancer pain[11,12] but there is insufficient clinical trial evidence for efficacy of treating cancer-related pain with TENS."[16]

Other physical treatments, including acupuncture, are covered later in this chapter in "Complementary and Alternative Medicine Approaches."

Functional-Capacity Evaluation

Individuals with chronic pain may be required to provide documentation of the extent of the injury or illness for purposes of work continuation, reassignment, or qualification for disability benefits. The *American Medical Association* has established a rating system that provides guidelines for quantifying the degree of disability present. However, many conceptual and practical issues are involved in classifying persons with chronic pain conditions.[17] Many clinicians treating pain require that other qualified professionals complete functional-capacity evaluations when asked to make work-related capacity decisions for individuals with chronic noncancer pain.

Psychological Treatments

Below are some of the psychological treatments utilized for treating chronic pain. A combination of psychological and medical treatments is usually more effective than unidimensional treatment for an individual's complex chronic pain problems.

Behavioral Therapies

Operant conditioning or contingency management involves changing the environment for the purpose of modifying behaviors. Behaviors are elicited by stimuli in the environment and are influenced by both their antecedents and consequences. Reinforcement increases behaviors and can be used to change behaviors.

An example of the use of contingency management for a person with chronic pain is observing the attention that is given in response to his or her pain behaviors. If family members pay special attention to the individual when he or she groans or lies down during the day, the person with pain may be inadvertently reinforced to display pain behaviors. As such, pain behaviors and disability tend to increase over time. In this instance, the focus of the response to the patient by individuals in the environment could be changed to giving the patient attention for active engagement, such as performing exercises during the day or going to work.[18]

Contingency management requires careful thought and a plan tailored for the individual. Family members or significant others may need to be involved. Contingency management can be used effectively to help patients increase their exercise and activity level.[18]

Psychophysiologic Techniques

Psychophysiologic techniques, such as relaxation and biofeedback, are directed toward helping the patient become aware of his or her ability to exert some control over physiologic processes of that he or she is not normally aware (e.g., muscle tension, skin temperature, respiration). Biofeedback uses feedback from a device or computer to give information to patients about their progress. Electromyography biofeedback is directed toward relaxing the muscles, which is particularly important in chronic pain conditions. Patients with low back or cervical pain tend to tense muscles around the site of their pain condition, bracing against it. This often causes increased pain due to muscle fatigue.

Biofeedback is also used in myofascial pain and temporomandibular joint syndrome. In addition to alleviating pain from reducing muscle tension, biofeedback can be used to increase peripheral skin temperature, causing dilation of vessels. This process can be helpful in the treatment of some types of headaches.[18]

The outcome of biofeedback research is generally positive, especially when combined with relaxation training. Individuals with migraine and/or tension-type headaches show a 56% success rate with temporal pulse amplitude biofeedback training.[18] A meta-analysis of biofeedback for headache found all biofeedback methods were effective for chronic headaches.[19] A combination of relaxation and thermal biofeedback are effective for recurrent migraines, while relaxation and/or EMG biofeedback may be appropriate as an adjunct or stand-alone therapy for recurrent tension headache.[20]

Relaxation Techniques

Relaxation techniques are a form of physiologic self-monitoring. Two popular procedures are progressive muscle relaxation and autogenic relaxation. Progressive muscle relaxation is a procedure that involves alternate tensing and relaxing of various muscle groups in sequence. This form of muscle relaxation is often coupled with diaphragmatic breathing and is helpful for patients who are unaware of their level of muscle tension.

Autogenic techniques involve repeating phrases subvocally (e.g.,

"My right hand feels heavy, warm, and comfortable.") and focusing the patient in a meditative manner as he or she is reclined or sitting quietly in a chair with eyes closed. Guided imagery can be used to focus the patient on changing reactions to his or her painful sensations, or to distract from painful experiences. Relaxation differs from hypnosis in that hypnosis involves a suggestion of pain relief and is generally thought to be a more concentrated form of relaxation. Relaxation and imagery have been found to reduce acute pain and procedural pain in patients with cancer pain.[20] Hypnosis will be discussed later on in this chapter in "Complementary and Alternative Medicine Approaches."

Cognitive-Behavioral Therapy

Cognitive-behavioral therapy (CBT) combines cognitive techniques with behavioral techniques. Cognitive techniques include changing distorted thoughts, such as "My pain is getting worse and will never get any better." Patients learn to observe their thoughts and how they affect their emotions and subsequent behaviors. Interventions are directed at changing the patient's thoughts to ones that are more realistic and engender positive coping behaviors.

Coping skills training includes identifying the patient's primary ways of coping with pain and changing those skills if they are not in the best interest of the patient's functioning. An example might be changing the patient's wishful thinking (passive coping) to seeking social support, increasing activities, or gaining more information about a problem (active coping).

Behavioral techniques that are commonly used in CBT are the psychophysiologic techniques (e.g., relaxation, imagery) discussed in the previous section and increasing appropriate activity, including pacing, problem-solving, and stress management. In addition, maladaptive behaviors are identified and targeted for change.[18]

CBT is an active therapeutic approach in which the therapist helps the patient set goals for treatment and engages the patient in completing homework in between sessions. CBT can help individuals with chronic pain focus and change their reactions to painful sensations, decrease negative emotional responses, and increase functioning. Advantages of CBT include a relatively short time course (usually 6–12 weeks), its evidence-based procedures and demonstrated effectiveness, and its applicability to a variety of pain-related difficulties (e.g., depression, anxiety) encountered by patients with chronic pain conditions. Meta-analysis of randomized clinical trials shows the efficacy of CBT and

■ **Table 6.1**

Randomized controlled evidence for
multimodal mind-body approaches for pain.

Type of Pain	Evidence for Efficacy
Chronic low back pain[20,21]	Multimodal approaches combining stress management, coping skills training, cognitive restructuring, relaxation therapy,[20] pain intensity, pain-related interference, health-related quality of life and depression[21]
Rheumatoid and osteoarthritis[20]	Multimodal approaches Cognitive-behavioral therapy, educational/ informational approach
Migraine headache [20]	Thermal biofeedback, relaxation
Tension headache[20]	Electromyography (muscle) biofeedback
Surgical pain (delivered presurgically) [20]	Hypnosis, imagery, relaxation
Invasive medical procedure pain [20]	Multimodal approaches may be helpful when used as an adjunct
Adult cancer pain[5]	A-level evidence: patient education and hypnosis
	B-level evidence: cognitive-behavioral coping skills (distraction and cognitive restructuring)
	Psychotherapy and structured support

psychological interventions as part of a multimodal approach to the treatment of chronic pain.[20,21,22]

A review of randomized controlled trials on mind–body therapies for managing pain found multimodal approaches effective. Table 6.1 summarizes some of these studies.

Psychosocial Interventions

Family Therapy and Family Interventions

Chronic pain can affect all family members. Family therapy focuses on the family unit and can change the patterns of behavior that are maladaptive. Family therapy should be considered when one or more family members exhibit behaviors that encourage maladaptive coping of the patient, if the family is overwhelmed by other difficulties, or if the patient is a child.

Educational Interventions for Families

Some educational interventions for families have been shown to be helpful, especially for families with patients with cancer. One target of such interventions is the patient and family barriers to adequate pain management described by the National Institutes of Health Consensus Statement.[23] These barriers are the following:

- Belief that pain is inevitable in cancer
- Belief that nothing can be done for cancer pain
- Fear of addiction and dependence on opioids
- Fear that drugs will lose their effectiveness
- Fear that reporting pain will exclude the patient from clinical trials or cancer treatments
- Failure to mention pain to providers
- Lack of adherence to treatment regimens
- High cost of medications and treatments
- Cognitive impairment hindering symptom assessment

Decreased pain has been found for cancer patients when education is directed toward alleviating these barriers, compared with those who received standard pain information.[24] Research shows that incongruence in beliefs about pain and pain experience between patients and caregivers results in the following:

- Poorer psychological functioning
- Poorer interpersonal functioning
- Lower quality of life
- Increased anger
- Increased fatigue
- Higher levels of caregiver strain[25]

Coping Skills Training for Couples

Coping skills training generally involves a combination of education, cognitive-behavioral skills, and relaxation training. Keefe et al.[22] trained partners of people with cancer in how to use cognitive behavioral pain-coping skills to assist their loved one toward the end of life. This line of research uses the patient's social milieu to improve pain coping and control.

Couples, Sexuality, and Pain

Couples often experience sexual problems after the onset of pain. Very little research has been conducted in this area. Patients with pain frequently experience the following:

- Decreased libido
- Decreased physical arousal
- Dyspareunia
- Postcoital pain

Pain and physical difficulties because of disability or illness can also impede a couple's usual sexual practices. These problems can affect relationships (e.g., satisfaction, intimacy), as well as identity (e.g., decreased feelings of femininity or masculinity). In addition, some medications used to treat pain or depression can cause sexual dysfunction. Prolonged use of opioids and antidepressants (most notably selective serotonin uptake inhibitors) can cause loss of libido and sexual disturbances in men (e.g., inability to attain or maintain an erection) and women (e.g., infertility, amenorrhea).

In evaluating patients with sexual dysfunction or difficulties, listening and asking questions concerning sexual functioning are significant parts of treatment. Many therapeutic modalities can be used to improve sexual dysfunction, including behavioral therapy, cognitive behavioral therapy, couples therapy, and sex therapy. Asking about sexual dysfunction is important because it can reveal treatable medical causes, such as low testosterone levels in men.

Group Therapy and Support Groups

Different types of therapy can be delivered in groups of 5–10 individuals and can range from coping-skills groups to support groups formed and led by persons with medical conditions. Mental health professionals (psychiatrists, psychologists, or social workers) generally lead therapeutic groups. These groups are usually psycho-educational or cognitive-behavioral in format and have been shown to be efficacious in increasing coping with chronic pain.

Patient-led support groups vary in effectiveness; some organized support groups provide emotional support and practical suggestions for members; others may focus more on limitations due to pain, dissatisfactions with the medical system, or other reinforcements for pain and dysfunction, all of which may perpetuate disability. In addition, a number of listservs and chat rooms are devoted to persons with various types of medical difficulties, including chronic pain conditions. The accuracy of information obtained from these sites varies, and patients should be critical of information they obtain through these methods.

Spiritual/Religious Support

Faith-based practices are important for many patients as a source of coping, support, and comfort in facing difficult situations and terminal illness. Patients with terminal illness may have existential questions and concerns best answered by a leader of their faith practice. Spiritual and religious beliefs often help patients make sense of their situations and serve as a guide for their future behaviors. Supportive members of faith communities may provide needed social support and/or assistance with tasks of daily living (e.g., grocery shopping). Clinicians may not understand the practices or beliefs of a particular patient, and patients may be hesitant to discuss how faith-based support is helpful to them. To the extent that religious and spiritual beliefs and practices can increase the patient's positive coping, facilitation of this process should occur.

Although a large body of research has been conducted on prayer and physical and mental health, few studies have been conducted on prayer and chronic pain. One study investigating the religious and spiritual practices of orthopedic patients with chronic pain found the following:

- Poorer physical health was related to private spiritual practices.

- Pain duration was associated with less forgiveness and less support from a religious or spiritual community.

- Poorer mental health was related to lack of forgiveness, feeling punished and abandoned by God, lack of daily spiritual experiences, little support from a religious community, and not being religious or spiritual.

- Pain, and interference due to pain, were not related to higher levels of religion or spirituality.[26]

Complementary and Alternative Medicine (CAM) Approaches

The National Center for Complementary and Alternative Medicine, a division of the National Institutes of Health, defines complementary and alternative medicine (CAM) as a "group of diverse medical and health care systems, practices, and products that are not presently considered to be a part of conventional medicine."[27]

Complementary medicine means that the practice is used with conventional medicine, such as music therapy used to soothe a patient after surgery. Alternative medicine is defined as practices that are used instead of conventional medicine, such as using herbal preparations as a treatment for rheumatoid arthritis, instead of drugs recommended by a doctor who practices conventional medicine.[27]

CAM interventions are divided into the following categories by the National Center for Complementary and Alternative Medicine:

- **Alternative medical systems** (e.g., Ayurveda, traditional Chinese medicine)

- **Mind-body interventions** (e.g., meditation, prayer)

- **Biologically-based therapies** (e.g., herbal products, vitamins)

- **Manipulative and body-based methods** (e.g., chiropractic or osteopathic manipulation, massage)

- **Energy therapies** (e.g., use of electromagnetic fields, biofield therapies such as Reiki and therapeutic touch)

Prevalence of Complementary and Alternative Medicine Practices

Americans are using many forms of CAM, and usage is growing. Consider the following statistics from the 2007 National Health Interview Survey conducted by the National Center for Health Statistics.[28]

- Approximately 38% of adults and 12% of children in the U.S. use some form of CAM.

- The most common CAM products used by American adults are natural, nonvitamin, nonmineral products (e.g., products from herbs and enzymes). Deep breathing and meditation are the second and third most practiced CAM modalities for American adults.

- Four of the top five conditions for which CAM modalities are most often used are chronic pain conditions and include:
  - Back pain
  - Neck pain
  - Joint pain
  - Arthritis pain

Mind-Body Interventions

The most studied mind-body interventions are *relaxation*, *meditation*, *imagery*, *biofeedback*, and *hypnosis*. Some of these are more studied and integrated into allopathic, or "conventional," medicine. Two of the more common interventions used for pain within the mind-body category are hypnosis and meditation. Massage, relaxation, and biofeedback are discussed in "Physical Manipulations" and "Psychological Treatments."

Hypnosis

Hypnosis is a state of deep relaxation that involves selective focusing, receptive concentration, and minimal motor functioning.[11]

Hypnosis has also been shown to do the following:

- Reduce chronic pain
- Reduce disability
- Improve postsurgical pain[20]
- Improve recovery time from surgery[20]

A review of controlled prospective trials of hypnosis in the treatment of a variety of chronic pain conditions found that hypnosis was more effective than attention, physical therapy and education.[29] However, a meta-analysis of hypnotic treatment for pain found that hypnosis was no more or less effective than relaxation techniques.[30]

Meditation and Mindful-Based Stress Reduction

There are a variety of meditative practices, many of which derived from Eastern culture or religious practices. *Mindfulness-based stress reduction (MBSR)* is a modern variant of meditation that has been applied to stress reduction. MBSR purports to change the experience of negative emotions by cultivation of an acute, moment-to-moment awareness of thoughts and feelings. A nonjudgmental attitude toward these thoughts and feelings is learned. This awareness is taught through regular meditative practice. Unlike many other meditative practices, MBSR has been studied for patients with chronic pain[31,32] and cancer.[33]

MBSR has been shown to improve the following:

- Chronic pain[31,32]
- Low back pain[31,32]
- Coping with pain[31,32]

- Stress[34]

- Mood[35]

- Immune system markers in patients with breast and prostate cancer[33]

Mindfulness-based art therapy, a combination of mindfulness practices and art therapy, has been shown to reduce psychological distress and improve the quality of life for patients with breast cancer.[36,37]

Biologically Based Therapies

Herbal Products

Many herbal products purport to relieve pain. A complete review can be found in the Clinical Tools section of **www.PainEDU.org.** Five of the top 10 herbal remedies in the United States are marketed to relieve pain. They are presented in Table 6.2.[38]

Herbal preparations are not subjected to the regulatory processes of other drugs, and therefore, a paucity of studies that assess their efficacy and safety exists. There are some well-controlled studies that, on the whole, document the limited efficacy of herbal treatments for pain relief.[38] However, clinicians should know what their patients are taking and ask about herbal preparations in a nonjudgmental manner.

■ Table 6.2
Herbs Marketed to Relieve Pain

Herb	Uses	Safety/Adverse Reactions
St. John's Wort (Hypericum perforatum)	Used for depression, anxiety, headache, muscle and nerve pain	■ Adverse effects: insomnia, anxiety, fatigue, headache. Is probably safe when used appropriately ■ May interact with drugs with serotonin, triptans, opioids, HIV drugs, digoxin, warfarin, oral contraceptives, chemotherapy, albuterol

■ **Table 6.2**
Herbs Marketed to Relieve Pain (continued)

Herb	Uses	Safety/Adverse Reactions
Echinacea (Echinacea purpura)	Used for migraines, dyspepsia, pain, dizziness, respiratory infection, wound healing	■ Adverse effects: allergic reaction, nausea, stomach pain, diarrhea, dizziness ■ May interact with acetaminophen, immunosuppressive therapy
Feverfew (Tanacetum parthenium)	Used for migraine	■ Adverse effects: headaches, ulcers, gastrointestinal upset ■ May interact with anticoagulants
Ginger	Used for nausea, gastrointestinal upset, thermal burns, topical analgesic	■ Generally safe when used appropriately. ■ Adverse effects: increased bleeding risk
Ginseng (Panax quinquefolius)	Used for memory, depression, headaches, fatigue	■ Adverse effects: anxiety, insomnia, headache ■ May interact with other drugs: nonsteroidal anti-inflammatory drugs, antipsychotic drugs, hormones, monamine oxidase inhibitors, immunosuppressants, opioids, alcohol

Manipulative and Body-Based Methods

Acupuncture

Acupuncture began in ancient China approximately 2,500 years ago. Its primary purpose according to Chinese philosophy is to assess and rebalance the life force of the individual. This life force is known as qi (pronounced "chee"). Qi is located on meridians of the body.

Stimulation of certain points on the meridians with small-gauge needles rebalances qi in the body. [39]

Western physicians have adopted forms of acupuncture, including pressure applied with the finger (acupressure), with low-frequency electrical current (electroacupuncture), or at points on the ear (auricular). [39,40,41]

The evidence is considered strong for the efficacy of acupuncture in postoperative pain and chemotherapy nausea and vomiting. [42] A meta-analysis found evidence that acupuncture is effective for pain relief for low back pain over sham acupuncture and no additional treatment. [43] Two reviews for cancer patients found the following:

- Pain relief

- Increased mobility

- Reduced cancer treatment-related pain

- Reduced muscle and bladder spasms

- Reduced vascular problems [44,45]

Literature reviews on the efficacy of acupuncture for short-term acute and for chronic pain are equivocal overall, since well-controlled studies are rare and long-term studies are lacking. [46] Empirical studies are difficult to accomplish for a number of reasons, including the absence of standardized treatments for certain conditions. Additionally, many practitioners of acupuncture do not believe the scientific methods of Western medicine are appropriate to study the efficacy of acupuncture.

Drawing on a scientific rationale of trigger point or electrical stimulation therapy, acupuncture is generally recommended for conditions that involve somatic pain. Adverse effects of acupuncture are bleeding and pain at the needle site. It is contraindicated for patients with thrombocytopenia, coagulopathy, or neutropenia. [40] Limitations of acupuncture include the possibility of infection if sterile precautions are not taken. In addition, some practitioners are overzealous about the effects of acupuncture and may promise more relief than is generally expected from any one treatment for acute or chronic pain. Properly practiced, acupuncture is considered safe and is an alternative or adjunct to conventional symptomatic treatments. [39,46]

Chiropractic or Osteopathic Manipulative Techniques

Chiropractic or osteopathic manipulation involves movement of the spine. They are used to reduce muscle tension and/or to place the patient's spine in proper alignment.

Limited evidence from systematic reviews supports chiropractic treatment for musculoskeletal conditions.[47] Osteopathic manipulative treatment has been found to be helpful in the treatment of chronic pain,[48] especially in reducing medication use and decreasing the need for physical therapy.[49] More research needs to be accomplished before these techniques can be recommended for the majority of patients with musculoskeletal pain.

Energy Therapies

Energy therapies involve manipulating the patient's energy to revive the energy flow in the body to enhance health. Energy is generally manipulated without touching the patient (e.g., therapeutic touch, Reiki, Qigong). Bioelectromagnetic-based therapies, such as the use of pulsed fields or magnetic fields are also in this category.[27]

There is not enough evidence about these therapies to recommend them. However, there are no known risks to these treatments.

Online Self-Management

Individuals with chronic pain and cancer pain are routinely looking online for information about their conditions.[50] Self-management takes a more active approach, using the Internet to deliver interventions that can promote positive health behaviors and offer support and self-management tools.

painACTION (*www.painACTION.com*) is an individually-tailored self-management site for patients with chronic pain. Site development was partially funded with NIH grants. Efficacy trials found that exposure to the intervention increased coping self-efficacy, increased use of social support, increased use of relaxation, and decreased pain catastrophizing.

PHARMACOLOGIC OPTIONS FOR THE MANAGEMENT OF PAIN

Non-opioid Analgesics

Acetaminophen

Acetaminophen has analgesic and antipyretic properties similar to that of aspirin, without the anti-inflammatory effect. Acetaminophen is a common treatment of mild to moderate pain and is often the recommended first-line analgesic therapy for the treatment of osteoarthritic pain.

Its mechanism of action is not well-defined, although it is thought to be associated with the nitric oxide cycle. Acetaminophen does not interfere with gastric mucosa protection or platelet aggregation. However, _doses in excess of 4 g per day should be avoided in all patients_ to minimize the risk of potentially serious liver toxicity. There has been recent controversy about the lack of public awareness with regard to potential risks of acetaminophen overdose. The Food and Drug Administration held a meeting in June 2009, a joint panel of the Drug Safety and Risk Management Advisory Committee, the Non-prescription Drugs Advisory Committee, and the Anesthetic and Life Support Drugs Advisory Committee. The panel recommended that a "black box" warning be issued for prescription medications that combine acetaminophen with another drug. The panel additionally voted to decrease the recommended daily maximum, and single adult dose maximum as well. Whether or not these recommendations are put into common practice remains to be seen.

Patients with chronic alcoholism and/or severe liver disease can develop hepatotoxicity even at therapeutic doses; therefore, care should be taken when prescribing acetaminophen in these patient populations. Clinicians should also be extremely vigilant when managing warfarin therapy in patients taking acetaminophen, as it can cause potentiation of the anticoagulant effects of warfarin.

Acetylsalicylic Acid

Acetylsalicylic acid, or aspirin, can sometimes be as effective as other non-opioid analgesics in relieving pain. Aspirin is commonly used to treat minor to moderate types of pain, including arthritic conditions, where its anti-inflammatory effect (similar to other non-steroidal anti-inflammatories) would be of benefit. Gastrointestinal disturbances (usually upper gastrointestinal) and bleeding due to platelet aggregation inhibition are the most common adverse effects seen with aspirin therapy. Although one of the oldest non-opioid analgesics and considered to be a member of the class of non-steroidal anti-inflammatory medications, the exact mechanism of aspirin is still unknown.

Because of the possible association with Reye's Syndrome, aspirin should be avoided in children younger than age 12 years with acute viral illness, particularly varicella, or influenza-like conditions. Aspirin should also be avoided by patients with peptic ulcer disease or poor kidney function because this medication can aggravate both conditions. Aspirin should also avoided in patients taking blood-thinning medications (anticoagulants), such as warfarin, because of an increased risk of bleeding.

Aspirin hypersensitivity may occur and can present with two distinct clinical pictures:

- In one presentation, the patient develops a respiratory reaction, with rhinitis, asthma, or nasal polyps.

- In another, smaller subset of patients, anaphylactoid symptoms may occur, such as urticaria, rash, hypotension, and shock within minutes of ingestion.

Nonselective Nonsteroidal Anti-inflammatory Drugs

Nonselective non-steroidal anti-inflammatory drugs (NSAIDs) are used primarily for treatment of mild to moderate pain and provide additive analgesia when combined with opioids prescribed for more severe pain conditions or inflammatory pain conditions. NSAIDs work by inhibiting the enzyme cyclooxygenase, which catalyzes the conversion of arachidonic acid to leukotrienes and prostaglandins, which are known to sensitize nociceptors near the location of the pain.[51] In contrast to opioids, NSAIDs have a distinct ceiling effect for analgesia—that is, increasing the dose beyond a certain threshold does not increase analgesia (but can increase toxicity). NSAIDs do not produce physical or psychological dependence.

NSAIDs are particularly good for bone pain and incident pain, or the type of pain that is provoked by activity (e.g., walking). All types of pain may respond to NSAIDs; however, visceral pain is probably less responsive than somatic pain, and neuropathic pain is often unresponsive.[52]

Although NSAIDs are useful for treating pain, patients should be carefully monitored for adverse effects, including renal impairment, bleeding, gastric ulceration, and hepatic dysfunction. Some less common side effects include confusion, precipitation of cardiac failure, pedal edema, and exacerbation of hypertension.

Extreme caution should be used when prescribing NSAIDs in patients who have any of the following risk factors:

- A history of gastric or duodenal perforation
- Peptic ulcer disease
- Concomitant use of anticoagulants (e.g., warfarin, heparin)
- Concomitant use of corticosteroids
- Prior history of long duration of use of NSAID therapy
- Advanced age

The optimal strategy for providing analgesia without gastrointestinal toxicity remains to be determined. Concomitant ulceroprotective treatment—for example, proton pump inhibitors or misoprostol—may be prescribed in high-risk patients. Although nonacetylated salicylates, choline-magnesium-trisalicylate, and salsalate appear not to alter platelet function significantly and are often used in this situation, clinical experience suggests that these medications are not as effective as the NSAIDs at relieving pain.

Cyclooxygenase-2 Inhibitors

Research has shown that there are actually two relevant isoforms of cyclooxygenase, COX-1 and COX-2. COX-1 is present in many tissues, including the gastrointestinal tract and platelets, whereas COX-2 is present primarily in inflamed/injured tissue and kidney. Thus, inhibition of COX-2 is likely the primary mechanism of action of NSAIDs, whereas inhibition of COX-1 is the mechanism of some of the major toxicities of NSAIDs: gastrointestinal ulceration, bleeding and platelet dysfunction. Agents that selectively inhibit COX-2 appear to relieve pain and inflammation without significant gastrointestinal or platelet disturbance. However, the analgesic efficacy of COX-2 inhibitors has not been proven to be superior to traditional NSAIDs. Indeed, with the current swirl of controversy surrounding cardiovascular risks that exists today with selective COX-2 inhibitors, these drugs should be used in appropriate patients who either are not at increased risk for complications, or in whom typical NSAIDs are not indicated due to risk factors such as those mentioned previously.

Opioid Analgesics

A Systematic Approach to the Use of Opioids in the Treatment of Chronic Pain

Opioids play an important and omnipresent role in the treatment of moderate to severe acute and chronic pain. In patients with acute pain, such as postoperative pain, opioids are utilized as the first-line treatment at least 98% of the time. Opioids are also recognized by many as the cornerstone of managing moderate to severe sub-acute and chronic cancer pain. Although their long-term safety and efficacy in chronic non-cancer pain patients continues to be debated, they also frequently play a role in management of this type of pain as well. Opioid analgesics are considered to be a mainstay in the treatment of moderate to severe pain that does not respond to non-opioids alone, because they are effective, are fairly easy to titrate, and have a favorable risk-to-benefit ratio. They are often combined with non-opioids because this permits using a lower dose (i.e., *opioid dose-sparing effect*).

Opioids can exhibit their analgesic effects by acting on both peripheral and central mu, kappa, and delta opioid receptors, which inhibits the transmission of nociceptive input from the periphery to the spinal cord, activates the inhibitory pathways that modulate transmission, and alters limbic system activity. Recent research expands the traditional view and shows that opioids may also work peripherally in areas of inflammation. Evidence also bears out that because responsiveness varies in individuals, a patient who has failed with one opioid should be treated with another to investigate greater efficacy.

Opioid analgesics are typically classified according to the receptors to which they bind, and are categorized as follows:

- Pure agonists
- Agonist-antagonists
  - Partial agonists
  - Mixed agonist/antagonists
- Pure antagonists
- Other
  - Tramadol

Pure agonists include the following:

- Codeine
- Dihydrocodeine
- Fentanyl
- Hydrocodone
- Hydromorphone
- Levorphanol
- Meperidine
- Morphine
- Methadone
- Oxycodone
- Oxymorphone
- Propoxyphene

These opioids are classified as *pure agonists* because they bind to the mu opioid receptor, do not have a ceiling effect for analgesia, and do not interfere with the effects of other opioids in this class when prescribed simultaneously. Side effects of full agonists include constipation, sedation, nausea and vomiting, mental clouding, addiction, myoclonus, pruritus, sweating, urinary retention, and respiratory depression.

Partial agonists (e.g., buprenorphine) bind with only partial efficacy at the opioid receptor. They have a ceiling effect for analgesia (e.g. NSAIDs) and may produce a withdrawal syndrome when administered to physically dependent patients.

Mixed agonists/antagonists include butorphanol, nalbuphine, and pentazocine. Unlike full agonists, these opioids block opioid analgesia at the mu opioid receptor, or are neutral at this receptor while simultaneously producing analgesia by activating another opioid receptor (kappa). Agonist/antagonists should not be prescribed with full agonists because doing so could lead to symptoms of withdrawal and increased pain.[9] Although the agonist/antagonists were initially thought not to cause addiction, experience has revealed the opposite. The agonist/antagonists thus have a limited role, if any, in pain management.

Pure antagonists, such as naloxone and naltrexone, are administered for prevention or reversal of opioid effects.

Tramadol is a useful agent that is unique in that it has a dual mechanism of action. Tramadol acts as a weak agonist at the mu opioid receptor, but also inhibits reuptake of norepinephrine and serotonin, like a tricyclic antidepressant. Both properties are necessary for its full analgesic activity. Tramadol is typically used for mild to moderate pain and can be used up to 400 mg per day, given as 25–100 mg every 4–8 hours as needed. Tramadol does not appear to produce tolerance, and although it can be addictive, this is much less common than with the other opioids. Tramadol is not an NSAID and does not share the NSAID liabilities of antiplatelet effect and gastrointestinal complications. Because of its tricyclic-like properties, tramadol should be used only with great caution in patients already on these agents. Also, tramadol can precipitate seizures, so it should be used with great caution, if at all, in patients with a history of seizures, brain metastases, or other risk factors for seizures.

The manufacturer of tramadol and the FDA notified health care professionals in May 2010 of changes to the warnings section of the prescribing information for tramadol. The strengthened warning information emphasizes the risk of suicide for patients who are addiction-prone, taking tranquilizers or antidepressant drugs, and also warns of the risk of overdosage.

Many primary care clinicians are reluctant to prescribe opioids for patients in pain outside of the most controlled of situations (e.g., when the patient is a hospital inpatient). This phenomenon is common, and accepted by clinicians *and* patients, resulting from a variety of factors:

- Clinicians who are not experts in the field of pain management may have had little **training** in the area of pain management beyond treatment of the short-term management of acute pain.

- Clinicians *and* patients may have **fears about becoming addicted or dependent** upon opioids, and have questions about these issues that go unanswered, and further propagate those fears and concerns.

- **Negative media coverage** about high profile opioid overdoses fuels additional public uncertainty at both the prescriber and patient level.

- Clinicians have fear of **regulatory scrutiny** and investigation if they prescribe these medications on a regular basis.

The easiest solution for the primary care clinician might seem to be to avoid the use of opioids when treating chronic pain altogether, and utilize alternative measures that exclude their use. In reality, that solution is likely an unrealistic and untenable solution, as the incidence of chronic pain is seemingly rising on an annual basis, and opioids remain an important, if not the hallmark component of a pain treatment plan. In fact, there is an outcry for *more effective* management of chronic pain than we currently achieve today, including a patient's right to demand it.

Despite concerns about opioid prescribing, primary health care providers remain the frontline practitioners faced with treating the most common kinds of chronic pain, such as back pain, arthritis pain, headache pain, and other common types of musculoskeletal pain. Beyond education directed towards primary health care providers about the pathophysiology of these common types of pain and its appropriate treatment, there have been many valuable contributions made by experts about the issues surrounding the responsible, safe and effective use of opioids when appropriate.

Experts in the field of pain management have suggested using common medical approaches and paradigms, similar to those used as part of routine clinical practices for other medical conditions. This can help allay some fears and concerns on both sides of the "opiophobic fence." It has the potential to improve the confidence level of clinicians to use opioids when they are the appropriate choice for the treatment of patients with chronic pain.

The term "universal precautions" originated from an infectious disease model that addressed an approach to patients when there was a deficiency of significant risk assessment information. Past behavior or practices were not reliable indicators of safe and reasonable approaches, especially with at-risk patients. In 2005, Gourlay, Heit, et al., proposed a *universal precautions*[53] approach to the use of opioids in the pain patient. The intention of the authors was to offer a structured, rational approach to pain patients and serve "as a guide to start a discussion within the pain management and addictions communities. They are not proposed as complete but rather as a good starting point for those treating chronic pain. As with universal precautions in infectious diseases, by applying the following recommendations, patient care is improved, stigma is reduced, and overall risk is contained."

These *universal precautions* for opioid use include the following 10 steps:

1. **Make a Diagnosis with Appropriate Differential** Along with other steps to arrive at a diagnosis for the cause of the patient's pain, address any comorbid conditions, including probable substance use disorders and other psychiatric illness.

2. **Psychological Assessment Including Risk of Addictive Disorders** A complete inquiry into past personal and family history of substance misuse is essential to adequately assess any patient. A sensitive and respectful assessment of risk should be done with available tools, and should not be seen in any way as

diminishing a patient's complaint of pain or reliability. Patient-centered urine drug testing (UDT) should be discussed with all patients regardless of what medications they are currently taking. Those found to be using illicit or un-prescribed licit drugs should be offered further assessment for possible substance use disorders. Those refusing such assessment should be considered unsuitable for pain management using controlled substances.

3. **Informed Consent**   The health care professional needs to educate the patient about the proposed treatment plan with opioids, including anticipated benefits, foreseeable risks, and concerns at a level appropriate to the individual patient.

4. **Treatment Agreement**   The expectations and obligations of both the patient and the treating practitioner need to be clearly understood. The format of this agreement can be verbal or written. Along with informed consent, the agreement should clearly identify responsibilities of both the clinician and the patient, monitoring for compliance plans, and any other important information that needs to be discussed.

5. **Pre- and Post-Intervention Assessment of Pain Level and Function**   Initiation of opioid therapy for patients in this setting should be considered a "trial" of therapy by both the clinician and patient. Without prior assessment of pain level and function, it would be impossible to measure progress.

6. **Appropriate Trial of Opioid Therapy +/– Adjunctive Medication**   Opioids may or may not be the first treatment of choice, and will most likely be used with other adjunctive medications. At this point, it is important to monitor the success or failure of the therapeutic trial with opioids.

7. **Reassessment of Pain Score and Level of Function**   Regular reassessment of the patient is critical to support continuation or discontinuation of the therapy.

8. **Regularly Assess the Four "A"s of Pain Medicine** Routine assessment of analgesia, activity, adverse effects, and aberrant behavior will help to direct therapy and support pharmacologic options taken.[54]

9. **Periodically Review Pain Diagnosis and Comorbid Conditions, Including Addictive Disorders** It is important to assess changes in the patient's condition and behavior. These need to be considered as dynamic phenomena.

10. **Documentation** Careful and complete documenting of the initial evaluation and each follow-up is both medico-legally indicated, and in the best interest of patients and clinicians. Thorough documentation can reduce medico-legal exposure and risk of regulatory sanction. A rule of thumb to remember is: if you do not document it, it did not happen.

Utilizing universal precautions for all patients who are appropriate candidates for opioid therapy has the potential to unify treatment plans, allow for unbiased application of treatment standards and monitoring, and can reduce the under-treatment of pain when opioids are part of the indicated solution.

Short-Acting and Long-Acting Opioid Preparations

Opioids may be classified according to whether they are short-acting or long-acting. *Short-acting opioids* include codeine, hydrocodone, hydromorphone, oxycodone, meperidine, and fentanyl (available for transmucosal use as a lollipop or buccal tablet). Short-acting agents are characterized by a relatively short onset of action (30–60 minutes) and relatively short duration of action (2–4 hours). Short-acting opioids are used generally for patients with mild to moderate pain, intermittent pain, or breakthrough episodes that are superimposed on constant background pain.

Other opioids may be characterized as *long-acting* by virtue of their intrinsic pharmacokinetic properties (e.g., methadone, levorphanol) or by virtue of their incorporation into a slow-release delivery system (e.g., controlled-release morphine, controlled-release oxycodone, transdermal fentanyl). Long-acting opioids are generally characterized by a slower onset of action, but a relatively long duration, and are therefore used on a round-the-clock basis for patients with constant background pain. Most patients with cancer pain end up on a long-acting opioid on a fixed-dose schedule for background pain with a short-acting opioid for breakthrough pain. Maximizing the use of long-acting opioids in this setting enhances adherence and affords patients the advantages of more consistent pain relief, increased sleep, decreased episodes of medication taking, and generally improved satisfaction. Although many clinicians have extended this treatment philosophy to individuals with chronic noncancer pain, the long-term advantages and disadvantages of these various approaches to opioid analgesia have not been systematically studied.

Abuse-Deterrent Formulations of Opioids

Along with the unparalleled benefits of opioids in managing pain, are the issues surrounding prescription opioid abuse, with rates approaching crisis levels. The possibility of abuse, addiction, or diversion of opioids is something that every clinician needs to consider when prescribing them. Regulatory agencies' approach to dealing with these issues has consisted of monitoring prescriptions, which some consider forces health care providers into a fearful corner when it comes to consideration of prescribing an opioid. This has often resulted in decreased comfort to prescribe opioids for the treatment of chronic pain, depending on certain patient characteristics, despite the appropriateness, or public outcry, for better management of pain.

Fueled by media attention, the issue seems to be worthy of concern. Indeed, even in secondary school students, the numbers can be intimidating; 20% of 7th–12th graders use prescription drugs non-medically,[55] with a significant amount of those medications being prescription opioids. The sources of abused or diverted opioids are quite varied, and can include:

- People with valid prescriptions
- Theft from the manufacturer, distributor, or pharmacy
- Theft of prescription forms from clinicians

- Theft or sale from the patient for whom the opioid was prescribed
- The Internet
- Drug dealers

Although opioids are often abused by the route that they were intended to be administered (e.g., orally), there is a significant amount of abuse after alteration or extraction of the active ingredient has taken place. In light of these facts, along with the diverse routes of availability, pharmaceutical companies manufacturing opioids have invested a large amount of resources towards the development of a number of different approaches to resist or deter abuse and misuse.

These *abuse-resistant or abuse-deterrent* formulations especially target techniques that are devoted to doubling or tripling doses, by extracting active ingredients out of the original formulation, allowing either an alternate route of administration (e.g., intravenous, smoking, or snorting), or concentration and increased potency of the opioid. In fact, the ability to extract the opioid out of a sustained-release opioid formulation can yield a very significant amount of abusable substance.

The abuse-deterrent strategies will generally work in one of two ways:

- Combining the active opioid along with another compound, like an opioid antagonist such as naloxone, to counteract the opioid effects if taken in large enough quantities, therefore decreasing its attractiveness for use by "blocking the high."
- Utilizing various compounding approaches designed to thwart the "hacking" of the medication. These include the use of physical barriers, or making it difficult to separate the delivery compounds from the active one, thereby making the opioid unsuitable for alternate forms of consumption (e.g., intravenous injection, smoking, or snorting).

The solution to curbing abuse of prescription opioids is a multifaceted one. These include a concerted effort of clinician education about appropriate patient assessment and selection; improved dialogue between health care providers and regulatory agencies about opioid prescription; improved patient education about safe practices; and close monitoring of patients perceived to be at a higher risk of abuse, misuse or addiction.

Abuse-deterrent opioid formulations may play a significant role in the approach to curbing prescribed opioid abuse and misuse.[56] They have the potential to provide opioids when appropriate, while limiting abuse and misuse, as well as its consequences. These abuse-deterrent formulations are intended to help to reduce the public health burden of prescription opioid abuse, and will also make it easier for clinicians to prescribe them when they are the appropriate choice for managing chronic pain. After validation of their ability to live up to expectations, they may become the new generation of opioids, and make non-deterrent formulations of opioids obsolete.

Appropriate Dosing of Opioids

An equianalgesic chart should be used when changing from one opioid to another, or from one route of administration to another. It is important to remember that the doses listed on equianalgesic charts are just estimates and can vary; the optimal dose for any individual patient is always determined by careful titration and appropriate monitoring. Equianalgesic charts show the oral and intramuscular (IM) doses of opioids that are equivalent to 10 mg of IM morphine. Because few studies exist comparing intravenous (IV) doses of different opioids, the American Pain Society[58a] recommends that IV doses be based on two assumptions: (1) that half the IV dose will give the same peak effect as a single IM dose and (2) IV infusions or repeated small boluses and IM total dosage will be equal when calculating the 24-hour requirements, because IM doses are eventually absorbed.

When a new drug is considered, the equianalgesic chart shows approximate equivalents between the new and old drug. The total dose of each opioid over 24 hours should be recorded, with separate calculations made for parenteral and oral doses of the same opioid if both forms are used. Each 24-hour total should be divided by the equianalgesic dose for that opioid and route, thereby converting the dose into equianalgesic dose units that are each equivalent to 10 mg of IM morphine. The equianalgesic dose units for all drugs should be added. The dose of the new drug can be found by multiplying the sum of the dose units obtained above by the equianalgesic dose for the new drug and route.[58a]

The equianalgesic dose conversion charts are derived mainly from single-dose analgesic studies and may not apply to chronic dosing. *The American Pain Society Principles of Analgesic Use in the Treatment of Acute Pain and Cancer Pain*[58a] indicate that dose changes for patients on high doses of opioids can be accomplished in stages by first implementing a partial conversion to minimize the risks of serious miscalculation (e.g. withdrawal, severe pain, overdose). For example, a patient with an infusion being changed to an oral preparation might have his or her infusion decreased by 50%, with the remaining 50% of the opioid requirement provided by an oral formulation. Reassessment of this strategy can be made after 24 hours. The half-life of opioids must also be taken into consideration when changing patients to different opioids. Estimates of doses vary widely depending on the half-life of the initial and replacement opioid, sometimes resulting in doses several times the original dose. In cases where the difference between severe pain from underestimating the conversion dose is coupled with safety concerns about overestimating the conversion dose, hospitalization for dose conversion is appropriate.

Routes of Administration of Opioids

The *oral* route of administration should be used first. This route is most convenient and cost-effective. It is a myth that *parenteral* administration of opioids is more effective at relieving pain than *oral* administration. *Effectiveness* (how well it works) must be distinguished from *potency* (how many milligrams it takes). *Oral* opioids are less potent than *parenteral* opioids—that is, higher doses of *oral* compared with *parenteral* opioids are required to produce the same degree of pain relief because of the first-pass metabolism of opioids in the liver. This has nothing to do with effectiveness—both routes work equally well at *equianalgesic* doses. However, the *parenteral*, *intramuscular* (IM), *intravenous* (IV), and *subcutaneous* (SC) routes may be required when the *oral* route is unavailable, rapid titration of opioid dose for severe pain is required, or the *oral* or *transdermal* opioid dose has become so high that only *parenteral* opioids can be conveniently administered. Because the ratio of *oral* to *parenteral* equianalgesic dosages differs among opioids, conversion charts are generally necessary when transitioning a patient from one opioid regimen to another. Liquid forms of opioids can be used when patients have trouble swallowing. Also, a number of liquid opioid preparations are fairly well-absorbed *sublingually* and come in various potencies (e.g., morphine, methadone), thus obviating the need for *parenteral* doses in patients who cannot swallow (e.g., esophageal cancer).

Fentanyl lozenges can be used *transmucosally* in patients with breakthrough pain who are unable to swallow or absorb medication. These fentanyl lozenges have the most rapid onset of action of any nonparenteral opioid. A recently approved rapid-onset (15 minutes) short-acting (60 minutes) *buccal* preparation of fentanyl received approval in 2009 for the management of breakthrough pain in patients with cancer who are already receiving and who are tolerant to opioid therapy for their underlying persistent cancer pain.

When *oral* opioids cannot be delivered secondary to unavailability of the *oral* route (e.g., nausea and vomiting), *rectal* and *transdermal* forms of administration should be considered. *Rectal* administration of opioids is possible but has a relatively slow onset of action and variable pharmacokinetics.[9] The *transdermal* fentanyl patch appears to be a safe and practical alternative to short-acting analgesics in the treatment of cancer pain. The unique pharmacokinetics of the *transdermal* system, including the prolonged time to peak analgesic effect, long elimination half-life, and skin depot concept, should be kept in mind when prescribing the system. A relatively new patient-controlled *transdermal* fentanyl patch is indicated for the short-term management of acute postoperative pain in adult patients requiring opioid analgesia during hospitalization.

IM injections should be avoided as a route of administration of opioid analgesia because of increases in pain that the injection can cause, unreliable absorption, and complications of IM shots (e.g., nerve injury, sterile abscesses).[9] In addition, oversedation can occur because of staircased doses given to achieve rapid analgesia. The *SC* route is a useful and underused mode of delivery of both isolated injections and long-term infusions. *SC* injections can provide rapid relief without the need for *IV* access. *SC* infusions can be used with patient-controlled analgesia pumps for long-term home use; patients can receive a continuous infusion plus boluses as needed. Generally a maximum of 2 ml per hour can be delivered this way; however, both morphine and hydromorphone can be concentrated to as high as 50 mg/ml, which covers nearly all situations. Induration or irritation at the infusion site can be a complication of *subcutaneous* infusion. *IV* patient-controlled analgesia requires IV access but does not have the volume limitations of *subcutaneous* infusions. In addition, opioid analgesia has more rapid onset when given *intravenously* versus *subcutaneously*. When IV patient-controlled analgesia is used, approximately 85% of individuals receive good to excellent pain control.[59]

Epidural and intrathecal administration of opioids directly to the spinal axis has gained widespread use because of its efficacy, especially for acute pain that has not responded to less invasive measures. However, side effects, such as pruritus, urinary retention, and delayed respiratory depression, are more common with these routes of administration. Opioids alone do not cause the same degree of hypotension from sympathetic blockade similar to that of local anesthetics because of their action only at opioid receptors, nor do they cause motor blockade that reduces patient mobility.[58a] However, opioids are generally used epidurally in combination with local anesthetics, due to the dramatic increase in analgesic efficacy of the combination; also, the combination allows relative reduction of opioid requirements and therefore opioid side effects.

Common Adverse Reactions

Constipation is commonly associated with opioid use, and all patients should receive prophylactic bowel therapy unless contraindicated. Increasing fluids, dietary fiber, exercise, and prophylactic medications may relieve constipation. Prophylaxis for opioid-induced constipation involves stimulants, such as senna derivatives, and stool softeners, such as docusate. It is important to note that dietary changes are rarely sufficient to counteract the constipation effects of opioids. If constipation develops, the cause and severity of the constipation should be assessed. A clinical history should include the time of the last two bowel movements, stool consistency, stool amount, use of laxatives, and other symptoms, such as nausea and distention.[52] The presence of fecal impaction, hemorrhoids, fissures, or an empty rectum should be established on physical examination. A good bowel movement every 3 days is a reasonable goal of treatment, depending on the patient's baseline.

After beginning an opioid analgesic, many patients complain of **sedation**. Although sedation usually abates in a few days, many patients report persistent sedation. To minimize sedation, administer opioids at the suggested starting doses, with lower doses for elderly or compromised patients, and then increase the opioid dose as necessary. When sedation develops, assess for other causes of sedation, including other sedating medications, sleep deprivation, systemic illness (e.g., hepatic or renal dysfunction), metabolic disturbances, and central nervous system pathology. The opioid dosage can be reduced if pain can be managed at a lower dose, although this is rarely useful because the patient likely uptitrated out of necessity for pain control. If the patient is using a significant dose of the opioid at bedtime to help with sleep, try nonopioid hypnotics (preferably ones with no morning carryover effect) to spare the total opioid burden. Administration of a co-analgesic (e.g., an NSAID) may allow opioid reduction. "Opioid rotation," or changing from one opioid to another, may reduce side effects. Opioid rotation may be necessary due to elimination of toxic opioid metabolites or to patients' idiosyncratic responses to different opioids. Psychostimulant medications are a useful symptomatic treatment for opioid-induced sedation and include caffeine, modafinil (200 mg every day to twice a day), dextroamphetamine (2.5–10 mg by mouth every day or twice a day), and methylphenidate (5–10 mg by mouth every day or twice a day).[58a] Stimulant medication generally should not be taken beyond 2p.m. to avoid interruption of sleep.

Opioids are thought to worsen the performance of psychomotor tasks because of their sedating and mental-clouding effects. As a result, some safety regulations restrict the use of opioids when driving or using heavy equipment.

A study was conducted to investigate the **psychomotor effects** of long-term opioid use in 144 patients with low back pain.[60] All subjects were administered two neuropsychological tests (Digit Symbol Substitution Test and Trail Making Test) before being prescribed opioids for pain (oxycodone with acetaminophen or transdermal fentanyl). Tests were then readministered at 90- and 180-day intervals. Test scores significantly improved while subjects were taking opioids for pain, which suggested that long-term use of short- and long-acting opioids does not significantly impair cognitive ability or psychomotor function. This supports the clinical impression that many patients who take opioids for pain over time adjust to the adverse effects of opioids, especially with regard to impaired cognition.[58a]

Nausea and vomiting are other common side effects associated with the use of opioids. Although drug-induced nausea is among the most common causes, other causes are possible (e.g., metabolic difficulties such as hypercalcemia or uremia, irritation of the gastrointestinal tract, pharyngeal lesions, brain metastases) and should be ruled out. New onset of nausea or vomiting in a patient who has been on an opioid for over a few weeks is not likely related to the opioid. Nausea and vomiting prophylaxis should be instituted in high-risk patients on initiation of opioid therapy. Treatment of nausea and/or vomiting should be aggressive if it occurs. To prevent opioid-induced nausea and vomiting in patients at risk, prescribe antiemetics with each opioid dose, at least until the patient's response seems stable and satisfactory. Some common anti-emetics prescribed to treat opioid-induced nausea and vomiting are dopamine-blocking agents (e.g., prochlorperazine, 10 mg; haloperidol, 0.5–1 mg; or metoclopramide, 10 mg, before each opioid dose), or 5-hydroxytryptamine 3 (5-HT3) receptor antagonists (e.g., ondansetron).

Opioids can sometimes cause **dysphoria or delirium**, as well as confusion, hallucinations, seizures, restlessness, and bad dreams. Opioid-induced delirium can often be resolved after a reduction of opioid, and sometimes by switching from one opioid to another.

Haloperidol, 0.5–2 mg by mouth every 4–6 hours, or other neuroleptic agents are effective symptomatic treatments.[9] It is useful to distinguish mental clouding caused by sedation from mental clouding caused by delirium. Psychostimulants may improve these symptoms in the former case but will usually worsen them in the latter.

Some patients develop **pruritus**, which can result from mast cell destabilization by the opioid and subsequent histamine release, or more likely, from central opioid effects on the brain or spinal cord. In many cases, the pruritus can be treated with a routine administration of long-acting, nonsedating antihistamines while opioid dosing continues. Although nalbuphine (an opioid agonist/antagonist) or naloxone may be effective, these agents should be used with caution to avoid precipitating withdrawal symptoms. Administration of an agonist/antagonist (e.g., butorphanol) has been shown to be very effective in treating opioid-induced pruritus without affecting analgesic efficacy. Sometimes switching opioids is the most pragmatic strategy for persistent opioid-induced pruritus.

Opioids occasionally cause multifocal **myoclonus**, which consists of sudden unexpected repetitive (but nonrhythmic) jerks of unrelated muscle groups throughout the body. This can be confused with "benign nocturnal myoclonus," a normal phenomenon consisting of a sudden jumping of seemingly the whole body during periods of drowsiness. Multifocal myoclonus is a characteristic feature of the opioid metabolite accumulation syndrome and should prompt concern, as it can progress to seizures. The approach consists of opioid rotation if possible; if not, the myoclonus can be suppressed with a number of agents (baclofen, valproic acid, clonazepam, gabapentin). Any medication that causes increased drowsiness can increase "benign nocturnal myoclonus," which should not arouse concern unless it is part of a progressive neurologic picture.

Urinary retention is sometimes caused by opioids but may be a more frequent problem associated with epidurally administered opioids. Urinary retention can be relieved with bethanechol or in the short-term with opioid antagonists (e.g. naloxone, naltrexone, or nalbuphine). It may be necessary to repeat doses to make certain that the bladder is completely empty, and sometimes catheterization of the bladder is necessary. Persistent urinary retention that is clearly due to an oral opioid should result in opioid rotation, along with measures to reduce opioid requirements.

Opioid-induced hyperalgesia (OIH) refers to a phenomenon whereby opioid administration results in a lowering of pain threshold, clinically manifested as apparent opioid tolerance, worsening pain despite accelerating opioid doses, and abnormal pain symptoms such as allodynia in a subset of patients on chronic opioid therapy. Typically, in patients suspected of having OIH, the clinical presentation includes increasing sensitivity to painful stimuli (hyperalgesia), and pain that becomes more diffuse, extending beyond the distribution of pre-existing pain. Currently, the consistency of the evidence for the occurrence of OIH in humans is unclear.[61]

Routine screening for opioid-induced **hypogonadism** is indicated for all patients on long-term opioid therapy. Opioid-induced hypogonadism is a common complication of opioid therapy in both men and women, occurring in the majority of patients in some studies. With the rising use of opioids for chronic pain, patient monitoring is increasingly important in order to manage possible endocrine complications. Symptoms may be subtle, and may include fatigue, mood changes, decreased libido, loss of muscle mass, and osteoporosis.

Respiratory depression is the most important opioid adverse effect. Opioids typically produce a concentration-dependent shift in the carbon dioxide response curve. When this shift becomes great enough, clinical expression of respiratory depression occurs, usually as a decrease in respiratory rate. Usually with clinically appropriate doses, compensation occurs, and respiratory rate does not decline. Tolerance to the respiratory effects of opioids usually develops quickly, and doses can generally be increased as necessary without concern. However, in the event of a cardiorespiratory event, a patient's response may be exaggerated due to the presence of opioid concentrations in the bloodstream. The point is that even in the absence of clinical signs, there may still be residual effects on respiratory reserve after tolerance develops, and this must be kept in mind with patients on opioid therapy. In cases where respiration is acutely compromised, the first priorities are, as always, establishing an airway and ventilating the patient. Consider using a dilute solution of naloxone (0.4 mg in 10 mL of saline), administered as 1-mL boluses every minute until the patient is breathing appropriately. Some patients are extremely sensitive to opioid antagonists. There is nothing more distressing to patients, family members, nurses, and physicians than overly aggressive administration of naloxone to a terminal patient resulting in a horrific withdrawal syndrome in the patient's last days or weeks. Patients remember opioid withdrawal forever—it is best avoided. Children and patients who weigh less than 40 kg should have 0.1 mg of naloxone diluted in 10 mL of saline to make a 10 mcg/mL solution, given at 0.5 mcg/kg every 2 minutes.[58a] Naloxone administration should not be given for altered mental status unrelated to opioid overdose.

Prescribing Considerations

Two major considerations are important when prescribing opioids: the *fear of regulatory and legal scrutiny and the fear of addiction*, which can ultimately contribute to the undertreatment of pain. Fears of sanctions by regulatory agencies are largely exaggerated. When prescribing guidelines are followed, investigations by regulatory agencies are unlikely.

Fear of Regulatory Scrutiny. The Federation of State Medical Boards of the United States has recognized the need for the use of opioids in pain management, and in 1998 published the *Model Guidelines for the Use of Controlled Substances for the Treatment of Pain*, which appears here:

1. *Evaluation of the Patient.* A complete medical history and physical examination must be conducted and documented in the medical record. The medical record should document the nature and intensity of the pain, current and past treatments for pain, underlying or coexisting diseases or conditions, the effect of the pain on physical and psychological function, and history of substance abuse. The medical record should also document the presence of one or more recognized medical indications for the use of a controlled substance. (*Many clinicians choose to use the*

SOAPP®, [Screener and Opioid Assessment for Patients with Pain], a brief paper and pencil tool, to facilitate assessment and planning for chronic pain patients being considered for long-term opioid treatment.[58b] The tool and accompanying scoring information can be downloaded from www.PainEDU.org.)

2. **Treatment Plan.** The written treatment plan should state objectives that will be used to determine treatment success, such as pain relief and improved physical and psychosocial function, and should indicate if any further diagnostic evaluations or other treatments are planned. After treatment begins, the physician should adjust drug therapy to the individual medical needs of each patient. Other treatment modalities or a rehabilitation program may be necessary depending on the etiology of the pain and the extent to which the pain is associated with physical and psychosocial impairment.

3. **Informed Consent and Agreement for Treatment.** The physician should discuss the risks and benefits of the use of controlled substances with the patient, persons designated by the patient, or the patient's surrogate or guardian if the patient is incompetent. *The patient should receive prescriptions from one physician and one pharmacy where possible.* The patient should agree to take medications only as prescribed. If the patient is determined to be at high risk for medication abuse or has a history of substance abuse, the physician may make use of a written agreement between physician and patient outlining patient responsibilities, including (1) urine/serum medication levels screening when requested, (2) number and frequency of all prescription refills, and (3) reasons for which drug therapy may be discontinued (e.g., violation of agreement).

4. **Periodic Review.** At reasonable intervals based on the individual circumstance of the patient, the physician should review the course of treatment and any new information about the etiology of the pain. Continuation or modification of therapy should depend on the physician's evaluation of progress toward stated treatment

objectives such as improvement in patient's pain intensity and improved physical and/or psychosocial function (e.g., ability to work, need of health care resources, activities of daily living, and quality of social life). If treatment goals are not being achieved despite medication adjustments, the physician should reevaluate the appropriateness of continued treatment. The physician should monitor patient compliance with medication use and related treatment plans.

5. *Consultation.* The physician should be willing to refer the patient as necessary for additional evaluation and treatment to achieve treatment objectives. Special attention should be given to those pain patients who are at risk for misusing their medications and those whose living arrangement poses a risk for medication misuse or diversion. The management of pain in patients with a history of substance abuse or with a comorbid psychiatric disorder may require extra care, monitoring, documentation, and consultation with or referral to an expert in the management of such patients.

6. *Medical Records.* The physician should keep accurate and complete records to include the following:
   - The medical history and physical examination
   - Diagnostic, therapeutic, and laboratory results
   - Evaluations and consultations
   - Treatment objectives
   - Discussion of risks and benefits
   - Treatments
   - Medications (including date, type, dose, and quantity prescribed)
   - Instructions and agreements
   - Periodic reviews

Records should remain current and be maintained in an accessible manner and readily available for review.

7. *Compliance with Controlled Substances Laws and Regulations.*
To prescribe, dispense, or administer controlled substances, the
physician must be licensed in the state and comply with applicable
federal and state regulations. Physicians are referred to the
Physician's Manual of the U.S. Drug Enforcement Administration and
any relevant documents issued by the state medical board for specific
rules governing controlled substances, as well as applicable state
regulations.

In addition, the Drug Enforcement Agency, along with a number
of other agencies, has issued a statement supporting the importance
of opioids in the management of pain. Clinicians can check these
guidelines, and others, in their communities.

*Documentation of the diagnosis, treatment and treatment outcome, as
well as periodic review*, is essential when prescribing opioids and serves
as protection in the event of investigation. An opioid agreement,
outlining the expectations of the patient and provider, can be used to
document informed consent and the responsibilities of patient and
provider. Such agreements often contain stipulations that the physician
be the only person to prescribe opioids and that the patient use one
pharmacy. These agreements outline appropriate use of opioids, side
effect information, and the type of behavior expected from the patient
(e.g., no requests for early refills, no changes in doses are made unless
the patient has been physically evaluated). They may also define
addictive behaviors and indicate the sanctions if the patient engages
in these behaviors. Family members and/or significant others may be
involved in these conversations so that they can learn more about the
risks and benefits of treatments with opioids. Physicians should review
any such agreements with their legal counsel before implementation,
because such agreements may have legal implications.

Fear of Addiction

Another fear that leads to the undertreatment of pain with opioids is
addiction. It is important that the clinician understands the distinction
between physical dependence, addiction, and pseudoaddiction, and
can convey this information to the patient and their family.

Physical dependence is a physiologic adaptation that occurs in patients receiving opioid analgesics (as well as other medications, including antiepileptics and certain antihypertensives). Physical dependence is characterized by the development of withdrawal symptoms when a medication is stopped or decreased abruptly and is expected in patients receiving opioid analgesics for more than a few days. Withdrawal can be avoided by tapering the dose when discontinuing treatment.

Addiction, on the other hand, is a chronic neurobiologic disease with genetic, psychosocial, and environmental influences. It is characterized by impaired control over drug use, compulsive use, continued use despite harm, and craving.

Pseudoaddiction is a term used to describe behavior that appears to be addictive, "drug-seeking" behavior, but is actually an effort to obtain pain relief by a nonaddicted patient who is not receiving adequate analgesia. Additional information on treatment of patients with comorbid substance abuse disorder is found in Chapter VII, in the section "Patients with Substance Abuse Problems." Although primary care practitioners often manage opioids for patients with chronic pain and cancer, they should not hesitate to refer patients to psychiatry, psychology, or pain management centers for consultation and/or evaluation and treatment.

Adjuvant Analgesic Agents

Adjuvant analgesic agents are a miscellaneous group of pain-relieving drugs whose primary indication traditionally is not for the treatment of pain. They are used to provide treatment for specific types of pain, and at times, to augment the analgesic effect of opioids and/or reduce the side effects of analgesics. Some of the most commonly used adjuvant drugs include corticosteroids, anticonvulsants, antidepressants, local anesthetics, neuroleptic agents, and hydroxyzine.

Corticosteroids

Corticosteroids are often used in palliative care, where they have a number of beneficial effects, including pain reduction, improved appetite, weight gain, antiemetic action, and mood elevation. Steroids are used in the treatment of neuropathic pain due to cord compression, brachial or lumbosacral plexus invasion, or peripheral nerve infiltration. Additionally, they are helpful in treating headache due to increased intracranial pressure, some types of arthritic pain, and pain after visceral obstruction.[52]

Dexamethasone, 12–24 mg/day, and prednisone, 30–100 mg/day, are the most commonly prescribed chronic regimens. Of course, the lowest dose that maintains benefit should be used; often, the best strategy is high initial doses followed by rapid tapering to the minimum effective dose. Beneficial effects of steroids tend to diminish after 2–3 months, and their use is therefore limited to patients with limited time left to live, or as a short-term treatment before the institution of other palliative measures.[52] Chronic use of corticosteroids produces weight gain, Cushing's syndrome, proximal myopathy, mental changes, and increased risk of gastrointestinal bleeding.[58a] NSAIDs should not, if possible, be used concomitantly with corticosteroids because of risks of gastrointestinal bleeding. Discontinuation of a corticosteroid should be made gradually to minimize the effects of a steroid withdrawal syndrome, which may occur due to adrenal suppression.

Anticonvulsants

Anticonvulsants are used for some neuropathic pain conditions to relieve lancinating or stabbing pain.[58] Anticonvulsants have the ability to suppress discharge in pathologically altered neurons, thus inhibiting neural hyperexcitability, which may be responsible for their usefulness in treatment of neuropathic pain conditions.

Gabapentin is a popular treatment choice because it is generally well-tolerated and serious side effects are extremely rare.[52] Gabapentin is indicated for treatment of postherpetic neuralgia, but also has been widely studied in treatment of other types of neuropathic pain. Unlike other anticonvulsants, gabapentin rarely causes hematologic or hepatic side effects. Effectiveness studies of gabapentin have shown wide variability in the dose (e.g., 100–3,600 mg) required to produce beneficial results. Consequently, gabapentin should be prescribed in low dosages initially, with titration as needed, and as tolerated.[52] Positive results are usually seen within 2 days, and therefore, upward titration may begin every other day, as needed.[52] Gabapentin is associated with the typical side effects of all central nervous system–acting drugs, including sedation, dizziness, and confusion.

Pregabalin is another anticonvulsant used to treat neuropathic pain. It was approved in 2004 for treatment of diabetic peripheral neuropathy and postherpetic neuralgia.

Other anticonvulsants used to treat pain include carbamazepine and phenytoin; however, the hematologic and hepatic side effects of these drugs have made them less popular than newer agents. Some studies have shown lamotrigine and topiramate useful in the treatment of neuropathic pain, but their higher side effect burden and requirement for prolonged titration have caused them to be a second choice for treatment. Finally, it should be highlighted that opioids are the main treatment choice for cancer pain, even neuropathic cancer pain, unless the pain can be controlled with adjuvants alone.

Tricyclic Antidepressants

Tricyclic antidepressants (TCAs), such as amitriptyline, imipramine, nortriptyline, and desipramine, are useful agents for neuropathic pain, cancer pain, and nonneuropathic pain with certain symptoms (e.g., insomnia, depression, or visceral spasm). Evidence suggests that tricyclic antidepressants suppress pain-signaling through local anesthetic-like effects at sodium channels in neural membranes. They also inhibit reuptake of norepinephrine, serotonin, and dopamine at synapses, which may increase their analgesic effects, as well as improve mood favorably.

Analgesic efficacy is best demonstrated for tricyclic antidepressants such as amitriptyline and nortriptyline, and duloxetine has recently been approved for the treatment of diabetic peripheral neuropathy, although it is not recommended in patients with a history of hepatic disease.

Common side effects include dry mouth, sedation, urinary retention, constipation, and orthostasis. They may also be associated with cardiovascular side effects, such as increased blood pressure and conduction blockade. They may also lower seizure threshold. Given that the efficacy of these agents is similar, choice of agent depends on the occurrence of side effects. Dosages for these agents are also comparable and should begin with 10–25 mg by mouth before bedtime and titrate upward as needed.[52] The usual beneficial dose for pain is 50–75 mg before bedtime; however, some patients may require 150 mg/day or more.[52] Although serum levels are not clinically useful for adjusting dosages, they are valuable for monitoring toxicity. It takes 2–4 weeks for analgesic effects to begin.

Topical Analgesics

Topical analgesics are targeted toward a specific area of pain. Typically, topical analgesics (e.g., lidocaine patch 5%, capsaicin) are applied directly onto the painful area. They act locally, so serum drug concentration is insignificant and systemic side effects are unlikely. Titration is not needed, and there are no drug interactions. Topical analgesics are used for both neuropathic and musculoskeletal pain. Capsaicin, derived from the active ingredient in chili peppers, is available over the counter and is widely used. Capsaicin depletes substance P from nerve terminals and is thought through this mechanism to decrease peripheral pain transmission. Clinical trials have reported efficacy in neuropathic pain, focal arthritis, and musculoskeletal conditions. These trials could not be adequately blinded (capsaicin stings), however, and the effect sizes seen were similar to those seen in unblinded trials.

NSAIDs are used topically around the world for localized pain; such use is less common in the United States, where these preparations must be custom compounded. However, many positive clinical trials and meta-analyses have confirmed the usefulness and safety of these preparations, apparently with a fraction of the systemic exposure of systemic NSAID treatment. Examples of such preparations include ibuprofen 5% and ketoprofen 20% cream.

Topical formulations are different from transdermal formulations. The application site for transdermal formulation is usually distant from the painful region and the formulation may have systemic effects, including serum drug concentration and possible side effects. Titration is needed, and drug interactions should be monitored for transdermal formulations.[60]

Several topical local anesthetics are available for use in pain treatment. Eutectic mixture of lidocaine and prilocaine is used to prevent acute procedure-related pain, such as that from venipuncture, circumcision, and skin biopsy. This medication is available as a cream and as a stick-on anesthetic disk. Although eutectic mixture of lidocaine and prilocaine is effective at reducing procedural pain, it must be left on for 30–60 minutes under an occlusive dressing before the procedure, which may be inconvenient. 4% liposomal lidocaine is another option for topical anesthesia to prevent acute procedural pain. The advantages of this preparation are that it seems to provide clinically relevant anesthesia at 60 minutes, comparable to that produced by eutectic mixture of lidocaine and prilocaine at 90 minutes, without requiring an occlusive dressing. These comparisons are based on a small number of generally poorly designed studies.

There are a number of topical anesthetic options for mucosal membranes. Dentists have used benzocaine and other agents effectively for oral anesthesia for generations. Lidocaine 2% jelly is available for coating instruments that are used for urethral or endotracheal intubation and for the topical treatment of urethritis-related pain.

Lidocaine patch 5% is the only *topical analgesic* approved by the Food and Drug Administration for postherpetic neuralgia. Unlike the topical anesthetics described previously, this patch does not produce anesthesia of the affected skin. With chronic use, systemic absorption also seems to be negligible. The lidocaine patch 5% should be applied directly to the most painful areas. Up to three patches may be used at a time, and they may be trimmed to conform to the affected area. The recommended dosage is to use the patch(es) for a maximum of 12 hours in a 24-hour period. The only significant side effect of the lidocaine patch 5%, in some cases, has been local skin irritation.

Neuroleptic Agents

Neuroleptic agents have been used as adjuvant analgesics for many decades; however, their role in the treatment of chronic pain is limited at present. Methotrimeprazine is the only neuroleptic with definite analgesic properties and is occasionally used for patients with opioid tolerance or side effects.[52] Common side effects of neuroleptics include sedation and hypotension. Prolonged use of phenothiazines is associated with tardive dyskinesia.[58a] Furthermore, extrapyramidal symptoms can occur, usually in younger patients, and can be treated with diphenhydramine.[58a] Other neuroleptics are used for the treatment of anxiety, psychosis, hallucinations, intractable insomnia, nausea, and vomiting.

Anxiolytics/Hypnotics

Hydroxyzine is an antihistamine, with anticholinergic (drying) and sedative properties, that is used to treat allergic reactions. In addition to its antihistamine effects, hydroxyzine has mild analgesic, antiemetic, anxiolytic, and sedative effects.

Hydroxyzine is usually prescribed at 25–50 mg by mouth or IM every 4–6 hours as needed (0.5–1 mg/kg for children).[58a] Although analgesic relief has been demonstrated after IM administration, it is not clear that oral administration produces any analgesic effects.[58a] As such, oral administration of hydroxyzine is mainly prescribed to relieve nausea or anxiety.

Cannabanoids

Cannabinoids are based on a chemical compound found in cannabis (marijuana). Tetrahyrocannabinol is one of the cannabinoids. None are approved for analgesia, but research into potential efficacy for pain management is ongoing.

Adjuvants for Bone Pain

Strontium (a radioisotope) and bisphosphonates are analgesic adjuvants used for metastatic bone pain. Radioisotopes work by delivering radiation to the bone. For example, one study demonstrated that a 10 m curie IV dosage of strontium was an effective adjuvant to local radiotherapy.[58a] Although they are effective for the pain of widespread bony metastases, they are complicated by bone marrow suppression.

Bisphosphonates are a class of agents originally used to treat hypercalcemia of malignancy that work by suppressing the process of bone resorption, which seems to be accelerated by malignancy. The most common bisphosphonate used for this indication is pamidronate, which has been shown to reduce skeletal events and pain in patients with metastatic breast cancer and other diseases associated with lytic lesions. Pamidronate is generally well-tolerated and is administered as 90 mg IV in 2 hours every 4 weeks.[58a] Another recently introduced agent is zoledronic acid, which has been shown to be effective not only in osteolytic lesions (e.g., breast cancer), but also osteoblastic lesions (e.g., prostate cancer). The relative roles of these different agents remain to be determined; treatment guidelines are available from the American Society of Clinical Oncology.

RATIONAL POLYPHARMACY AND PAIN MANAGEMENT

The American Society of Anesthesiologists Task Force published the following guidelines in *Anesthesiology* in 2004: *Acute Pain Management Practice Guidelines for Acute Pain Management in the Perioperative Setting: An Updated Report by the American Society of Anesthesiologists Task Force on Acute Pain Management.*

Part of these guidelines states that *"Whenever possible, anesthesiologists should use multimodal pain management therapy. Unless contraindicated, all patients should receive an around-the-clock regimen of nonsteroidal anti-inflammatory drugs (NSAIDs), cyclooxygenase-2 inhibitors (COXIBs), or acetaminophen. Dosing regimens should be administered to optimize efficacy while minimizing the risk of adverse events. The choice of medication, dose, route, and duration of therapy should be individualized."*

Analgesics exert their activity at various sites along the pain pathway. Thus, in theory, multimodal analgesia [i.e., the use of two or more agents with differing mechanisms or multiple modes of analgesia (e.g., local anesthetics and opioids)] increases the likelihood that pain signals will be interrupted and pain relieved. Research has shown that analgesics with differing mechanisms of action can have additive or synergistic effects through a variety of cellular mechanisms, allowing the use of lower doses of each agent than would be used during monotherapy. A multimodal approach to pain management has long been proposed for treatment of both acute and chronic pain. The

World Health Organization, the Agency for Healthcare Research and Quality (formerly the Agency for Health Care Policy and Research), and clinicians endorse the use of more than one agent with different mechanisms of action for the treatment of pain. The goal of multimodal therapy is to increase the efficacy of pain relief with enhanced safety and tolerability.

Below is a diagram by Gottschalk et al. depicting the different sites of action of many of the previously mentioned analgesics, portraying the idea that a multifocal approach could be beneficial.[62]

■ Figure 5

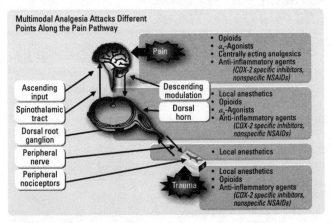

Multimodal analgesia attacks different points along the pain pathway.
Gottschalk A, Smith D. New concepts in acute pain therapy: preemtive analgesia. *Am Fam Phys* 2001;63:1979-1984.

Multimodal analgesia attacks different points along the pain pathway.[63]

The idea that multimodal therapy, or rational polypharmacy, should be applied toward effective pain management is actually not new. The logic is that, to most successfully treat pain, two strategies are beneficial:

1. Attempt to "attack" pain at as many points along the pathway as possible.

2. Minimize the dose of medications with high adverse effect profiles in concert with other medications. This should likely minimize the incidence of adverse effects.

As stated in the previous guidelines for acute pain management, when treating pain, all decisions should be made with respect to the individualized treatment for the patient. For more information, please refer to the appendixes for medications and dosing information.

INTERVENTIONAL OPTIONS FOR THE MANAGEMENT OF CHRONIC PAIN

The history of the application of interventional techniques in pain management dates back to 1901, when epidural injections for lumbar nerve root compression were reported.[64] Since then, substantial advances have been made in the administration of epidural injections, and many other interventional techniques have been described. Interventional techniques have been distinguished as the favored, and at times decisive, intervention in both the diagnostic and therapeutic management of chronic painful conditions.

Diagnostic and Therapeutic Blocks

Regional anesthesia refers to regional neural blockade for the purpose of blocking or modifying afferent or efferent neural conduction. Diagnostic, or differential, nerve blocks have been used to determine the source of the pain, differentiate local from central processes, identify nociceptive pathways, and differentiate between local and referred pain,[65] although there are important limitations to these approaches. For example, a sympathetic nerve block can determine whether the pain is sympathetically maintained, which would guide treatment decisions, but with a high false-positive rate. Diagnostic blocks are sometimes used to decide whether a neuroablative block would be effective, but their predictive value in this regard remains to be demonstrated. Local anesthetics and other agents can be infused via an indwelling catheter in the epidural space, or along peripheral nerves to provide analgesia for days to weeks. Local anesthetics with or without steroids can be injected into various structures to provide anti-inflammatory effects and pain relief. These techniques are useful in treating pain from joints, bursae, and spinal nerves.

Facet Joint Blocks

The facet joints of the spine can be anesthetized by fluoroscopically guided injections of local anesthetic, either into the target joint or onto the medial branches of the dorsal rami that supply them. The rationale for facet joint blocks is based on the observation that if a particular joint is determined to be the source of pain generation, long-term relief can be sought by directing therapeutic interventions at that joint. In managing low back pain, local anesthetic injection into the facet joints, or interruption of the nerve supply to the facet joints, has been accepted as the standard for diagnosis of facet joint mediated pain.

Trigger Point Injections

Trigger point injections are probably the most extensively used modality of treatment, not only by interventional pain physicians, but by all providers managing pain. Myofascial pain syndrome is a regional muscle pain disorder accompanied by trigger points. It has been described as a common phenomenon in multiple regions, including the spine. Myofascial trigger points are small, circumscribed, hyperirritable foci in muscles and fascia, often found within a firm or taut band of skeletal muscle. In contrast, nonmyofascial trigger points may also occur in ligaments, tendons, joint capsule, skin, and periosteum. Trigger points assist in the proper diagnosis of myofascial pain syndrome.

Neurolysis

Neurolytic agents (e.g. alcohol, phenol, and glycerol) injected around the nerve produces destructive changes in the nerve to decrease pain transmission. Other techniques to alter functioning of nerves include cryotherapy (cold) and radiofrequency (heat) lesions. Although these techniques can result in significant pain relief, complete destruction of the nerve can be accomplished only with surgical resection.[66] Neurolysis of the visceral ganglia can be used for visceral pain associated with cancer. Neurolytic techniques are also used to treat neuropathic pain. Neurolytic nerve blocks are generally reserved for intractable pain in the cancer setting, due to their inherent risks and the high rate of pain recurrence. Extreme consideration must be made when selecting patients for this technique, as it is ablative in nature and irreversible.

Interventional Techniques

Sympathetic blocks using regional anesthetic techniques and radio-frequency thermoneurolysis, neuromodulation with spinal cord stimulation, or peripheral nerve stimulation are often management options for reflex sympathetic dystrophy, and causalgia, also known as complex regional pain syndrome (CRPS) types I and II. Radiofrequency neurolysis is really an extension of a continuous regional sympathetic block or neurolytic block, providing long-term relief with added safety. Consideration of sympathetic blocks is to facilitate management of complex regional pain syndrome with analgesia, commensurate with a program of functional restoration and sympatholysis to provide unequivocal evidence of sympathetically maintained pain. Once it is established that sympatholysis is effective, it is important to repeat the procedure to determine whether an increasing duration of effect can be expected in any particular patient. If this is the case, these individual blocks may be all that are necessary to enable a patient to regain function. When sympatholysis completely relieves the symptoms and facilitates exercise therapy but is limited to its duration of effect, it is appropriate to consider a prolonged block using radiofrequency neurolysis. Radiofrequency has been described for lesioning of the cervical sympathetic chain, thoracic sympathetic chain, and lumbar sympathetic chain; in cases of complex regional pain syndrome I and II, as well as for neuropathic pain.

Implantable Technologies

Spinal cord stimulation and peripheral nerve stimulation are techniques that involve electrical stimulation of the spinal cord or peripheral nerves via an implanted pulse generator that delivers electrical signals to these structures. In the United States, the primary indications for spinal cord stimulation are failed back surgery syndrome. Patients experience a "buzzing" feeling that is associated with reduced pain intensity. These signals are thought to stimulate large afferent fibers and inhibit the noxious signals mediated by A delta and C-fibers.[66] Spinal cord or peripheral nerve stimulation appears to be most effective for individuals with chronic neuropathic pain, peripheral vascular disease, or chronic angina.

Implantable intrathecal pumps can deliver a continuous infusion of analgesic medications (e.g., morphine) directly to the spinal cord. Implantable pumps can be useful in the management of cancer pain or intractable chronic pain of noncancer origin. For a few patients, they may be used when the side effects of oral opioids are intolerable. Proper patient selection, as with all forms of pain management strategies, is critical for the success of implantable technologies.

REFERENCES

1. Lee MHM, Itah M, Yang GW, Eason AL. Physical therapy and rehabilitation medicine. In: Bonica JJ (ed). *The Management of Pain*. Vol 2. 2nd ed. Philadelphia, PA: Lea & Febiger; 1990:1769–1788.

2. Vasudevan S, Hegmann K, Moore A, Cerletty S. Physical methods of pain management. In: Raj PP, ed. *Practical Management of Pain*. Baltimore, MD: Mosby; 1992:669–679.

3. American Society of Anesthesiologists Task Force on Chronic Pain Management. Practice guidelines for chronic pain management: An updated report by the American Society of Anesthesiologists Task Force on Chronic Pain Management and the American Society of Regional Anesthesia and Pain Medicine. *Anesthesiology*. 2010; 112; 810-833.

4. Carlson AH. Hot & cold. Tried and true ice and heat modalities still prove effective for acute and chronic pain. *Rehabilitation Management*. 2007;20:32-33.

5. Miaskowski C, Cleary J, Burney R, Coyne P, Finley R, Foster R, et al. Guideline for the management of cancer pain in adults and children. APS Clinical Practice Guidelines Series, No. 3. Glenview, IL: American Pain Society (APS); 2005.

6. National Comprehensive Cancer Network. *NCCN Clinical Practice Guidelines in Oncology: Adult Cancer Pain*. (V.1.2010). National Comprehensive Cancer Network, Inc. http://www.nccn.org. Accessed July 30, 2010.

7. Mclean JP, Chimes GP, Press JM, Hearndon ML, Willick SE, Herring SA. Basic concepts in biomechanics and musculoskeletal rehabilitation. In: Fishman

SM, Ballantyne JC, Rathmell JP, eds. *Bonica's Management of Pain*. 4th ed. Philadelphia: Lippincott Williams & Wilkins; 2009:1294-1312.

8. Allen RJ, Wilson AM. Physical therapy agents. In: Fishman SM, Ballantyne JC, Rathmell JP, eds. *Bonica's Management of Pain*. 4th ed. Philadelphia: Lippincott Williams & Wilkins; 2009:1345-1356.

9. Jacox AK, Carr DB, Payne R, et al. Management of Cancer Pain, Clinical Practice Guidelines. No. 9. Rockville, MD: U.S. Department of Health and Human Services, Public Health Service, Agency for Health Care Policy and Research (AHCPR Publication No. 94-0592), 1994.

10. Field TM. Massage therapy effects. *Am Psychol*. 1998;53:1270–1281.

11. Monti DA, Yang J. Complementary medicine in chronic cancer care. *Semin Oncol*. 2005 Apr;32(2):225-231.

12. Ernst E. Musculoskeletal conditions and complementary/alternative medicine. *Best Pract Res Clin Rheumatol*. 2004 Aug;18(4):539-556.

13. Wilke DJ, Kampbell J, Cutshall S, et al. Effects of massage on pain intensity, analgesics and quality of life in patients with cancer pain: a pilot study of a randomized clinical trial conducted within hospice care delivery. *Hosp J*. 2000;15(3):31–53.

14. Chabel C. Transcutaneous electrical nerve stimulation. In: Loeser JD, Butler SH, Chapman CR, Turk DC, eds. *Bonica's Management of Pain*. 3rd ed. Philadelphia: Lippincott Williams & Wilkins; 2001:1842–1848.

15. Nnoaham KE, Kumbang J. Transcutaneous electrical nerve stimulation (TENS) for chronic pain. *Cochrane Database Syst Rev*. 2001;(3):CD003222.

16. Robb K, Oxberry SG, Bennett MI, Johnson MI, Simpson KH, Searle RD. A cochrane systematic review of transcutaneous electrical nerve stimulation for cancer pain. *J Pain Symptom Manage*. 2009 Apr;37(4):746-53. Epub 2008 Sep 14.

17. Robinson JP, Tait RC. Disability evaluation in painful conditions. In: Fishman SM, Ballantyne JC, Rathmell JP, eds. *Bonica's Management of Pain*. 4th ed. Philadelphia: Lippincott Williams & Wilkins; 2009:279-288.

18. Turk DC, Swanson KS, Tunks ER. Psychological approaches in the treatment of chronic pain patients-when pills, scalpels, and needles are not enough. *Can J Psychiatry*. 2008 Apr;53(4):213-223.

19. Martin PR, Forsyth MR, Reece J. Cognitive-behavioral therapy versus temporal pulse amplitude biofeedback training for recurrent headache. *Behav Ther*. 2007 Dec;38(4):350-363. Epub 2007 Sep 27.

20. Astin JA. Mind-body therapies for the management of pain. *Clin J Pain*. 2004 Jan-Feb;20(1):27-32.

21. Hoffman BM, Papas RK, Chatkoff DK, Kerns RD. Meta-analysis of psychological interventions for chronic low back pain. *Health Psychol*. 2007 Jan;26(1):1-9.

22. Keefe FJ, Abernethy AP, Campbell LC. Psychological approaches to understanding and treating disease-related pain. *Annu Rev Psychol.* 2005;56:601-630

23. National Institutes of Health. Symptom management in cancer: pain, depression and fatigue: State-of-the-Science Conference Statement. J Pain Palliat Care Pharmacother. 2003;17(1):77-97.

24. Oliver JW, Kravitz RL, Kaplan SH, Meyers FJ. Individualized patient education and coaching to improve pain control among cancer outpatients. *J Clin Oncol.* 2001;19(8):2206-2212.

25. Miakowski C, Zimmer EF, Barrett KM, Dibble SL, Wallhagen M. Differences in patients' and family caregivers' perceptions of the pain experience influence patient and caregiver outcomes. *Pain.* 1997;72(1-2):217-226.

26. Rippentrop EA, Altmaier EM, Chen JJ, Found EM, Keffala VJ. The relationship between religion/spirituality and physical health, mental health and pain in a chronic pain population. *Pain.* 2005;116(3):311-321.

27. National Center for Complementary and Alternative Medicine, National Institutes of Health. *Cam Basics: What is CAM?* Bethesda, MD: National Center for Complementary and Alternative Medicine; February 2007. NCCAM Publication No. D347. http://nccam.nih.gov/health/whatiscam/index.htm. Accessed July 1, 2010.

28. Barnes PM, Bloom B, Nahin R. CDC National Health Statistics Report #12. *Complementary and Alternative Medicine Use Among Adults and Children: United States, 2007.* December 10, 2008. http://nccam.nih.gov/news/camstats/ Accessed July 1, 2010.

29. Elkins G, Jensen MP, Patterson DR. Hypnotherapy for the management of chronic pain. *Int J Clin Exp Hypn.* 2007 Jul;55(3):275-287.

30. Jensen MP, Patterson DR. Hypnotic treatment of chronic pain. *J Behav Med.* 2006;29(1):95-124

31. Kabat-Zinn J, Lipworth L, Burney R. Four year follow-up of a meditation-based program for the self-regulation of chronic pain: treatment outcomes and compliance. *Clin J Pain.* 1987:27:466-475

32. Kabat-Zinn J, Lipworth L, Burney R. The clinical use of mindfulness meditation for the self-regulation of chronic pain. *J Behav Med.* 1985;8:163-190.

33. Carlson LE, Speca M. Mindfulness-based stress reduction in relation to quality of life, mood, symptoms of stress, and immune parameters in breast and prostate cancer outpatients. *Psychosom Med.* 2003;65:571-581.

34. Coker KH. Meditation and prostate cancer: integrating a mind/body intervention with traditional therapies. *Semin Urol Oncol.* 1999;17:111-118.

35. Carlson LE, Ursuiliak Z, Goodey E, Angen M, Speca M. The effects of a mindfulness meditation based stress reduction program on mood and symptoms of stress in cancer patients: 6-month follow-up. *Support Care Cancer.* 2001;9:112-123.

36. Monti DA, Peterson C. Mindfulness-based art therapy: Results from a two year study. *Psychiatr Times*. 2004; 2221:6663-6666.

37. Monti DA, Peterson C, Kunkel EJ, et al. A randomized controlled trial of mindfulness-based art therapy (MBAT) for women with cancer. *Psychooncology*. 2006 May;15(5):363-373.

38. Wirth JH, Hudgins JC, Paice JA. Use of herbal therapies to relieve pain: a review of efficacy and adverse effects. *Pain Manage Nurs*. 2005;6(4):145-167.

39. Yang J, Monti DA. Acupuncture and Chinese medicine. In: Monti DA, Beitman BD, eds. *Integrative Psychiatry*. New York:Oxford University Press, Inc.; 2010:127-158.

40. Deng G, Cassileth BR, Yeung KS. Complementary therapies for cancer-related symptoms. *J Support Oncol*. 2004 Sep-Oct;2(5):419-426.

41. Filshie J, Thompson JW. Acupuncture. In: Doyle D, Hanks NC, Calman K, eds. *Oxford Textbook of Palliative Medicine*. 3rd ed. New York: Oxford University Press, Inc.; 2004:410-424.

42. Staud R. Mechanisms of acupuncture analgesia: effective therapy for musculoskeletal pain? *Curr Rheumatol Rep*. 2007 Dec;9(6):473-481.

43. Manheimer E, White A, Berman B, Forys K, Ernst E. Meta-analysis: Acupuncture for low back pain. *Ann Intern Med*. 2005 Apr 19;142(8):651-663.

44. Filshie J, Redman D. Acupuncture and malignant pain problems. *Eur J Surg Oncol*. 1985 Dec;11(4):389-94.

45. Filshie J. Acupuncture for malignant pain. *Acupunct Med*. 1990;8(2):38-39.

46. Melchart D, Weidenhammer W, Streng A, et al. Prospective investigation of adverse effects of acupuncture in 97,733 patients. *Arch Intern Med*. 2004 Jan 12;164(1):104-105.

47. Ernst E. Manual therapies for pain control: chiropractic and massage. *Clin J Pain*. 2004 Jan-Feb;20(1):8-12.

48. Pujol LM, Herbert B. Integrative approaches to the management of chronic pain. In: Monti DA, Beitman BD, eds. *Integrative Psychiatry*. New York:Oxford University Press, Inc.; 2010:240-267.

49. Licciardone JC. The unique role of osteopathic physicians in treating patients with low back pain. *J Am Osteopath Assoc*. 2004 Nov;104(11 Suppl 8):S13-8.

50. Eng TR, Gustafson DH. US Department of Health and Human Services: Science Panel on Interactive Communication and Health; Office of Public Health and Science. *Wired for Health and Well-Being - The Emergence of Interactive Health Communication*. Washington, DC: US Printing Office; 1999.

51. Buvanendran A, Lipman AG. Nonsteroidal anti-inflammatory drugs and acetaminophen. In: Fishman SM, Ballantyne JC, Rathmell JP, eds. *Bonica's Management of Pain*. 4th ed. Philadelphia: Lippincott Williams & Wilkins; 2009:1157-1171.

52. Katz NP. Pain and symptom management. In: Kantoff PW, Carroll PR, D'Amico AV, et al, eds. *Prostate Cancer: Principles and Practice*. Philadelphia: Lippincott Williams & Wilkins; 2002:561–594.

53. Gourlay DL, Heit HA, Almahrezi A. Universal precautions in pain medicine: a rational approach to the treatment of chronic pain. *Pain Med*. 2005 Mar-Apr;6(2):107-12.

54. Passik SD, Weinreb HJ. Managing chronic nonmalignant pain: overcoming obstacles to the use of opioids. *Adv Ther*. 2000;17(2): 70-83.

55. McCabe SE, Boyd CJ, Young A. Medical and nonmedical use of prescription drugs among secondary school students. *J Adolesc Health*. 2007 Jan;40(1):76-83. Epub 2006 Oct 5.

56. Katz NP, Adams EH, Chilcoat H, et al. Challenges in the development of prescription opioid abuse-deterrent formulations. *Clin J Pain*. 2007 Oct;23(8):648-60.

57. Fischer B, Rehm J. Nonmedical use of prescription opioids: furthering a meaningful research agenda. *J Pain*. 2008 Jun;9(6):490-3.

58a. American Pain Society. *Principles of Analgesic Use in the Treatment of Acute Pain and Cancer Pain*. 4th ed. Glenview, IL: American Pain Society; 1999.

58b. Butler SF, Budman SH, Fernandez K, et al. Validation of a screener and opioid assessment measure for patients with chronic pain. *Pain*. 2004;112:65–75.

59. Ashburn MA, Ready LB. Postoperative pain. In: Loeser JD, Butler SH, Chapman CR, Turk DC, eds. *Bonica's Management of Pain*. 3rd ed. Philadelphia: Lippincott Williams & Wilkins; 2001:765–779.

60. Jamison RN, Schein JR, Vallow R, et al. Neuropsychological effects of long-term opioid use in chronic pain patients. *J Pain Sympt Manage*. 2003;26:913–921.

61. Zylicz Z, Twycross R. Opioid-induced hyperalgesia may be more frequent than previously thought. *J Clin Oncol*. 2008 Mar 20;26(9):1564.

62. Galer BS, Dworkin RH. *A Clinical Guide to Neuropathic Pain*. New York: The McGraw-Hill Companies; 2000.

63. Gottschalk A, Smith D. New concepts in acute pain therapy: preemptive analgesia. *Am Fam Physician*. 2001;63:1979–1984.

64. Cathelin, M. Mode d'action de la cocaine inject dons l'espace epidural par le proceda de canal sacre. *CR Soc Biol*. 1901.

65. Melton S, Liu SS. Regional anesthesia techniques for acute pain management. In: Fishman SM, Ballantyne JC, Rathmell JP, eds. *Bonica's Management of Pain*. 4th ed. Philadelphia: Lippincott Williams & Wilkins; 2009:723-754.

66. Govind J, Bogduck N. Neurolytic blockade for noncancer pain. In: Fishman SM, Ballantyne JC, Rathmell JP, eds. *Bonica's Management of Pain*. 4th ed. Philadelphia: Lippincott Williams & Wilkins; 2009:1467-1485.

VII.

Pain Management in Special Patient Populations

INFANTS AND CHILDREN

The myth that pediatric patients do not experience the same degree of pain as adults do was routinely taught to clinicians in training until fairly recently. The foundation of faulty logic was that infants and children had nervous systems that were not yet fully developed, and do not retain memories of their earlier years. Actually, recent animal studies show the opposite is true and that due to a stronger inflammatory response, along with decreased central inhibition, infants and children most likely deal with a higher level of pain than adults do. Indeed, it may be purely the lack of the ability to appropriately communicate the severity of pain that results in undertreatment of pain in this patient population.

Assessment of pain in this special population can be challenging, but is possible. Observational tools as well as physiologic parameters such as heart rate, respiratory rate, and oxygen saturation, have been shown to be valid means to assess the degree of pain that a child is feeling.

Tables 7.1 and 7.2 are two examples of the commonly used validated observational tools for assessment of pain in infants and children.

■ Table 7.1
CRIES Neonatal Postoperative Pain Scale[1]

(Crying, Required FiO2, Increased HR and BP, Expression, Sleepless)

	0	1	2
Crying	No	High-pitch, consolable	Inconsolable
Required FiO2 to maintain SaO2 at least 95%	No	<30%	>30%
Increased heart rate and blood pressure	No	11–20% increased	>20% increased
Expression	Calm	Grimace	Grimace and grunt
Sleepless	No	Frequent awakening	Constantly awake

Scores are added up to an assessment range of a 0–10 pain level.

■ Table 7.2
FLACC Scale[2]

(Face, Legs, Activity, Cry, and Consolability Scale)

	0	1	2
Face	No particular expression or smile	Occasional grimace or frown, withdrawn, disinterested	Frequent to constant quivering chin, clenched jaw
Legs	Normal position or relaxed	Uneasy, rest-, less tense	Kicking or legs drawn up
Activity	Lying quietly, normal position or relaxed	Squirming, shifting back and forth, tense	Arched, rigid or jerking
Cry	No cry (awake or asleep)	Moans or whimpers, occasional complaint	Crying steadily, screams or sobs, frequent complaints *(continued)*

■ **Table 7.2**
FLACC Scale[2] *(continued)*

	0	1	2
Consolability	Content, relaxed	Reassured by occasional touching, hugging, or being talked to, distractible	Difficult to console or comfort

Scores are added up to an assessment range of a 0–10 pain level.

Management of pain in the pediatric population should occur within a relationship among the treatment team, the child, and his or her parents or guardians. The parents or guardians usually end up being the single most important and passionate advocate for aggressive pain management in infants and children.

Effective treatment usually combines pharmacologic and nonpharmacologic interventions.

Nonpharmacologic interventions include several psychological techniques, such as imagery and relaxation training. Moreover, some practical techniques include minimizing unnecessary procedures and discussing procedures in an age-appropriate manner.

With respect to pharmacologic treatments, the medications used to treat pain in infants and children are similar to those used in adults. However, some special considerations are important. Aspirin and its derivatives should be avoided in patients with pain coexisting with any kind of viral syndrome-like symptoms who are younger than the age of 19, unless specifically indicated, due to the incidence of Reye's syndrome. Most analgesics and local anesthetics are metabolized through the liver, and in the first 6 months of life, the liver may be relatively immature and require dosage adjustments of medications to compensate for this immaturity. Newborn infants usually have a decreased glomerular filtration rate in the first week of life. Newborn infants also have a relatively higher percentage of body weight that is water, resulting in an increased volume of distribution.

Treatment interventions for children with cancer pain include analgesics, adjuvants, regional analgesia, chemotherapy, and radiation

■ **Table 7.3**

**Basic Principles of Pain Management
in Infants and Children**

- Neuroanatomic components and neuroendocrine systems are sufficiently developed to allow transmission of painful stimuli in the neonate and child.

- Pain in newborns and children is often unrecognized and undertreated. Neonates *do* feel pain, and analgesia should be prescribed when indicated during medical care.

- If a procedure is painful in adults, it should be considered painful in newborns, *even if they are preterm*.

- Compared with older age groups, infants and children may experience a greater sensitivity to pain and are more susceptible to the long-term effects of painful stimulation.

- Adequate treatment of pain may be associated with decreased clinical complications and decreased mortality.

- Sedation does not provide pain relief and may mask the child's response to pain.

- A lack of behavioral responses (including crying and movement) does not necessarily indicate a lack of pain.

- Severity of pain and the effects of analgesia can be assessed in the pediatric patient. Healthcare professionals have the responsibility for providing a systematic approach to pain management, including assessment, prevention, and treatment of pain in this patient population.

- Treatment should include the appropriate use of environmental, behavioral, and pharmacologic interventions.

- Environment should be as conducive as possible to the well-being of the child and family.

- Education and validation of competency in pain assessment and management for all clinicians are a professional responsibility and very important when it comes to caring for pediatric and adult patients.

therapy. It is important to note that most medications have not been tested in children, and therefore, prescribing medications to children should follow the World Health Organization approach. Acetaminophen is relatively safe for relief of mild pain, and can be administered orally or rectally.[3] Nonsteroidal anti-inflammatory drugs (NSAIDs) are not recommended for patients with cancer who also suffer from thrombocytopenia. When pain is moderate to severe, opioid analgesics are effective and should be administered orally whenever possible. Children should be administered "rescue" doses, particularly if they are receiving continuous infusion. Regular monitoring of side effects is important given that children are often unable to communicate side effects that they may be experiencing (e.g., pruritus, constipation).

Table 7.3 provides a good set of basic principles that should routinely be considered when treating and assessing pain in infants and children.

ELDERLY PATIENTS

Elderly patients with pain are another group of patients who are often understudied and undertreated. Despite the fact that the prevalence of pain increases with age, the use of analgesic medication declines.[4] The reasons for undertreatment are due to human error. Some include the following:

- Under-reporting of pain by patients due to accepting it as a consequence of aging

- Sensory impairments might hinder the patient's ability to communicate the degree and source of pain

- Public and clinician attitudes about aging and pain influence tendencies to treat

- Long-term care facilities consist of staff that may be less educated about pain management than those working in acute care facilities

- Cognitive impairment can interfere with an elderly patient's ability to complete pain assessment instruments and adhere to a prescribed treatment regimen

- Reluctance to prescribe opioids due to adverse effects, such as confusion or delirium

All elderly patients should be considered to be at increased risk for undertreatment of pain. Assessment of function is critical in assessing pain in elderly patients. The ability to perform activities of daily living is of paramount importance in elderly patients, as they may be solely responsible for their own care or the care of a spouse. Because depression and signs of chronic pain may frequently coexist, elderly patients may exhibit decreased socialization, which may go unrecognized, and they may further suffer from the inability to care for themselves.

The likelihood is that pain in elderly patients stems from one of three causes:

- A result of a **coexisting medical illness**

- A result of **aging** (e.g., spinal stenosis or osteoarthritis)

- As part of a **neuropsychiatric disorder**

Of course, there may be overlap, but this categorization usually helps to establish the best course of treatment. The treatment must obviously try to address the specifics of the causes.

Initial treatments for elderly patients with mild to moderate chronic pain have traditionally included acetaminophen and NSAIDs. Recently a significant amount of attention has been devoted to guidance on the use of pharmacotherapeutic agents in elderly patients with chronic pain. The American Geriatrics Society (AGS) published its first Clinical Practice Guidelines on management of persistent pain in older adults in 1998. In 2002, these guidelines were revised. In 2009 the guidelines were again revised,[5] providing the recommendations for new pharmacologic approaches. Because the most common strategy for managing persistent pain among older adults is through use of pharmacologic agents, and because this is also potentially the area of greatest risk, this updated guideline focuses on pharmacotherapy. *"The recommendations in this guideline represent the consensus of a panel of pain experts and were derived from a synthesis of the literature combined with clinical experience in caring for older adults with persistent pain.[5]"*

These guidelines recommend *"that acetaminophen be considered as initial and ongoing pharmacotherapy of patients with mild to moderate musculoskeletal pain, but—in a significant departure from the 2002 guideline—recommends that nonselective NSAIDs and COX-2 selective inhibitors be considered rarely, with caution, in highly selected individuals. The new guideline recommends that all patients with moderate to severe pain, pain-related functional impairment or diminished quality of life due to pain be considered for opioid therapy. The new guideline also provides new references and discussions regarding use and limitations of newer adjuvant, topical, and other drugs for recalcitrant pain problems.[6]"*

Addiction and tolerance to opioids seem, from clinical experience, to be significantly less of a problem in the elderly, whereas the risks of the adjuvant agents, such as mental status changes and falling, appear to be greater. Thus, the risk-to-benefit ratio may favor opioids over other agents in the elderly. Of course, this still remains a controversial issue. Due to differences in metabolism, some older patients appear to be more likely to experience opioid side effects, such as cognitive and neuropsychiatric dysfunction, than younger patients. Therefore, a slow titration schedule beginning with minimal doses might be preferable to more aggressive titration as in a younger patient.

Similarly, interventional treatment, such as spinal cord stimulation and intrathecal analgesia, although often perceived as invasive and risky, may actually be safer than long-term pharmacologic approaches for some elderly patients. Other treatment options include cognitive-behavioral therapy, physical therapy, and multidisciplinary treatment. Aggressive rehabilitation is particularly important in the elderly, who are particularly prone to rapid deconditioning and whose ability to function depends on fine degrees of conditioning. Clinicians should be careful not to undertreat pain in the elderly; treatment of pain in this population should be approached with patience and balance.

PREGNANT AND LACTATING PATIENTS

When possible, the use of nonpharmacologic treatments should be maximized for noncancer pain in pregnancy. These include judicious rest, pacing, various harnesses designed for pregnancy, ice and heat, and other physical therapy modalities. In general, NSAIDs are avoided. Acetaminophen is generally considered safe in clinical practice. Despite a dearth of data, opioids are widely used for severe pain during pregnancy and are considered relatively safe.

When there are questions with regard to safety it is important to consider consulting with the obstetrician-gynecologist before administering pain medication to a pregnant or lactating patient.

The Food and Drug Administration has created a categorization of drugs based on empirical findings and safety for use in pregnancy[7]:

Category A	Adequate, well-controlled studies in pregnant women have not shown an increased risk of fetal abnormalities.
Category B	Animal studies have revealed no harm to the fetus; however, there are no adequate and well-controlled studies in pregnant women. *Or* Animal studies have shown an adverse effect, but adequate and well-controlled studies in pregnant women have failed to demonstrate risk to the fetus. *Or* No animal studies have been conducted, and there are no adequate and well-controlled studies in pregnant women.
Category C	Animal studies have shown an adverse effect, and there are no adequate and well-controlled studies in pregnant women.

Category D	Studies in animals or pregnant women have demonstrated a risk to the fetus. However, the benefits of therapy may outweigh the potential risk.
Category X	Studies in animals or pregnant women have demonstrated positive evidence of fetal abnormalities. The use of the product is contraindicated in women who are or may become pregnant.

There are many problems with the current system of drug labeling and categories in pregnancy, however. There are very few drugs in category A and very few drugs in category X. In fact, 70% of drugs are category C, but not all category C drugs have the same level of risk. New pregnancy labeling soon to be implemented by the Food and Drug Administration will include summary of risk assessment, clinical considerations, and data, and, it is hoped, provide more detailed guidelines for safe use of medications in this special patient population.

RACIALLY AND ETHNICALLY DISPARATE PATIENTS

"Clearly, medical degrees do not confer immunity from conscious or unwitting acts of discrimination."[16]
—David B. Morris

The United States is increasingly racially and ethnically diverse. By 2050, if not before, the current U.S. "white majority" will be the minority.[8] The National Institutes of Health defines health disparities as "differences in the incidence, prevalence, mortality, and burden of diseases and other adverse health conditions that exist among specific population groups in the United States[9]."

Many researchers have investigated the role of race and ethnicity when studying the prevalence of pain and the burden of pain in the

United States. The majority of these studies have found a higher pain prevalence and higher pain burden for disparate populations. Studies have examined this in different settings including:

- Analgesic dosing in emergency departments and postoperative care units

    A classic example of this is the research on differences in analgesia for long bone fractures in an urban emergency department[10]

- Access to pharmacies that stock controlled substances in diverse communities

    Research in New York City and the state of Michigan demonstrated less access to pharmacies and pharmacies with adequate stocks of pain medication[11,12] in disadvantaged neighborhoods

- Incidence of joint replacement for arthritis

- Proportion of referrals for palliative care

In 2002, the Institute of Medicine (IOM) of the National Academies of Sciences published *"Unequal Treatment: Confronting Racial and Ethnic Disparities in Health Care."*[13] It reported that these disparities in pain assessment and treatment existed for all types of pain across the life span. A U.S. Department of Health and Human Services goal for improving the health for all Americans by 2010 was to eliminate disparities in health status.[14]

In 2009, *The Journal of Pain* published an article reviewing the progress in addressing the racial and ethnic disparities in pain. The authors reviewed research articles published between 1990 and early 2009, and concluded that although there has been a lot of attention paid to this concern, disparities continue to exist in the management of acute pain, chronic cancer pain, and palliative care.[15]

The many causes of these disparities can be summarized as three factors. *They all play an important role:*

- *Patient related.* An individual's culture and history, income, education, employment and language all play a large role in attitude and response to illness and medical treatment.

- **System related.** Systemic factors that are related to an increased burden of pain include access to health insurance coverage and access to health care practitioners and facilities.

- **Provider related.** Provider beliefs and expectations of patients, which may remain largely unchallenged throughout their education and training, can contribute to disparities.

Since the prevalence of pain has significant socioeconomic and health ramifications for the individual and society, more effort is needed to research and develop practices and policies designed to eliminate disparities in health care.

WOUNDED WARRIORS

Since 2001, with the deployment of U.S. military forces engaged in wars in Iraq and Afghanistan, there has been increased focus on the need for comprehensive policy and services for pain management for returning veterans. The Veterans Health Administration (VHA) Pain Management Strategy was developed in 1998, establishing pain management as a national priority.[17] This strategy has had many updates since then.[18]

A VHA National Pain Management Strategy teleconference in 2009, led by Robert D. Kerns, Ph.D., the National Program Director for Pain Management, presented these facts about veterans and pain[19]:

- As many as 50% of male VA patients in primary care report chronic pain.

- The prevalence may be as high as 75% in female veterans.

- Pain is among the most frequent presenting complaint of returning soldiers from Operation Enduring Freedom (Afghanistan) and Operation Iraqi Freedom, particularly in patients with polytrauma.

- Pain is among the most costly disorders treated in VHA settings.

Several factors make the experience of the troops returning from Iraq and Afghanistan different than the experience of troops in other wars:

- Advances in battlefield medicine and protective armor for the torso have led to more survival of injuries that would have been fatal in prior conflicts.

- Many of these injuries have been defined by the VHA as "polytrauma, two or more injuries to physical regions or organ systems, one of which may be life threatening, resulting in physical, cognitive, psychological, or psychosocial impairments and function disability." [20]

- Identification of a triad of three conditions found together: chronic pain, posttraumatic stress disorder (PTSD), and traumatic brain injury (TBI)[20]

- A force made up a large number of reserve and National Guard troops, who may have enlisted never expecting to find themselves in combat

- Long deployments and multiple deployments[20,21]

The problems experienced by these returning veterans (especially traumatic brain injuries, PTSD, and completed suicides) have garnered a great deal of attention and emphasis on the need for the VHA to expand its services. Clinicians who do not work for the VHA are also affected, as many veterans receive their health care at non-VA facilities. Most of these veterans have parents, spouses, and children who were significantly impacted by their deployment, and they struggle with a host of problems when their loved one returns home.

HOSPICE AND PALLIATIVE CARE PATIENTS

During the 1960s Dr. Cicely Saunders began the modern hospice movement by establishing St. Christopher's Hospice near London. It was the first program using modern pain management techniques to compassionately care for the dying. In the United States, demonstration projects assessed the cost-effectiveness of Medicare payment for hospice care beginning in 1979. By 1982, Congress had created a hospice benefit, and in 1986, the benefit became permanent.

The American Board of Medical Specialties officially recognized Hospice and Palliative Medicine as a medical specialty in 2006. Since that time, the field has grown rapidly. Hospice and palliative medicine specialists train to care for people when cure may not be a realistic or achievable goal. In many cases, these specialists are called upon to treat patients in moderate to severe pain, with incurable conditions, or near the end of their lives due to a terminal illness.

From a reimbursement perspective, insurers may cover many facets of palliative care as part of standard treatment. Most health insurances (including Medicaid and Medicare) cover hospice care in a bundled fashion when a physician and a hospice medical director certify that the patient is terminally ill, with 6 months or less to live.[22] It is important to note that this "certification" can be extended if the patient survives longer than six months.

The World Health Organization (WHO) defines palliative care as "An approach that improves the quality of life of patients and their families facing life-threatening illness, through the prevention, assessment, and treatment of pain and other physical, psychosocial, and spiritual problems."

The WHO underscores the principles that palliative care should strive to achieve the following goals:

- Provide relief from pain and other distressing symptoms.
- Affirm life and regard dying as a part of the life cycle.
- Intend neither to hasten or postpone death.
- Offer a support system to help patients live as actively as possible until death.
- Offer a support system to help the family cope during the patient's illness and in their own bereavement, including the needs of children.
- Use a team approach to address the needs of patients and their families, including bereavement counseling, if indicated.
- Enhance the quality of life that may also positively influence the course of a patient's illness.

Recent guidelines developed by the National Consensus Project for Quality Palliative Care were published in 2009.[23] This is how they describe palliative care:

> *"The goal of palliative care is to prevent and relieve suffering and to support the best quality of life for patients and their families, regardless of the stage of the disease or the need for other therapies, in accordance with their values and preferences. Palliative care is both a philosophy of care and an organized, highly structured system for delivering care. Palliative care expands traditional disease-model medical treatments to include the goals of enhancing quality of life for patient and family, optimizing function, helping with decision-making, and providing opportunities for personal growth. As such, it can be delivered concurrently with life-prolonging care or as the main focus of care."*

Both hospice and palliative care share the same philosophy of care with the intention of a smooth transition linking them together, even though they often have different basic structures. A palliative care program will coordinate patient care across multiple locations and providers. Palliative care programs generally address the physical, psychosocial, and spiritual needs and expectations of a patient with a life-threatening illness, *at any time during that illness, even if life expectancy extends to years*. Palliative care does not preclude aggressive treatment of an illness, and provides comfort to patients and their loved ones.

The goal of hospice care is usually *to keep pain and suffering of a person with a terminal diagnosis to a minimum, and not to cure the illness*. Provided in the patient's home or in hospice centers, hospitals, skilled nursing homes and other long-term care facilities, hospice is based on the belief that every person has the right to die pain-free and with dignity, with family and friends nearby, while making the end-of-life as comfortable as possible.

"Adequate relief of pain at the end of life is an ethical imperative… people are more likely to die after a long, protracted illness, and pain is a common comorbidity of these illnesses."[24] Pain can be both physical and existential. Cancer is often named as an illness with a likelihood of physical end-of-life pain, but other illnesses, such as HIV, multiple sclerosis, ALS, end stage renal disease, and heart disease, can also have pronounced pain. Pain assessment at the end of life can be a challenge. It can be hard to determine whether pain is due to the progression of the underlying disease, or is due to the treatment for the disease. The diagnostic challenges increase if the patient is a child, is cognitively impaired, or is not verbal.

From a treatment perspective, different routes of drug delivery may offer better choices with the end-of-life patient. These include:

- Oral

- Rectal

- Sublingual, transmucosal, or buccal

- Nasal

- Intravenous

- Spinal

- Topical

- Transdermal

Patients and their family members may have fears about addiction to pain medications in the end-of-life or palliative care setting. Additionally, some health care providers may question appropriate analgesic dosages, especially as they are increased and other medications are added. Therefore, patients and their families need education about pain management, and reassurance that their loved one will not become addicted. Patients should be encouraged to express their wishes about future care, including pain medication and possible tradeoffs with wakefulness.

Regulatory and legal concerns about prescribing pain medication are present for some clinicians in the end-of-life setting. These fears can be a major barrier to providing appropriate pain management. Fears of sanctions are generally exaggerated. In fact, the opposite problem has occurred multiple times in recent years: successful litigation against a clinician for failing to control pain at the end of life. A clinician prescribing opioids appropriately for cancer pain will almost never be investigated, although due to variability across communities in the U.S., local prescribing guidelines should be checked. Documentation of diagnosis and treatment, including the outcomes of opioid treatment, is essential and provides protection in the event of regulatory scrutiny. Read more about regulatory and legal concerns in the Opioid Analgesics section starting on page 153 .

Intractable pain or unmanageable adverse effects can often lead to incredible suffering. The pharmacokinetics of the opioids and other analgesics that are used to manage pain can sometimes be altered by organ dysfunction associated with the disease or dying process. In end-of-life situations, the clinician must weigh the burden of pain against the possibility of treatment hastening death. Sometimes sedation may even be a treatment option for intractable pain. The point is that this care needs to be provided with great consideration and planning.

Whether treating an incurable condition or providing end-of-life care, it is essential to provide as much information and support as possible to the patient, family members, and other loved ones, to assure that decision-making responsibility about making the patient as comfortable as possible is appropriately agreed upon and shared.

COGNITIVELY IMPAIRED PATIENTS

As mentioned previously, pain is a common phenomenon in the elderly patient population because the likelihood of these patients suffering from conditions such as cancer and arthritis problems is increased. Cognitive impairment is another condition with increased incidence in this patient population. Undertreatment of pain in this patient population is only compounded by the coexistence of cognitive impairment. Indeed, cognitive impairment may be responsible for preventing one of the single most important signs needed to treat pain—the ability to communicate suffering. This can make the accurate assessment of pain in those with severe cognitive impairment one of the most significant challenges in the field of pain management.[25] This also makes information available from family and caregivers invaluable.

Pain management in the absence of a detailed history can prove quite challenging. Although caregiver information is critical, it may be incomplete due to the lack of exhibition of normal pain behavior. Sometimes, the signs that cognitively impaired patients exhibit are not discrete or obvious, but may be the only clues available, including the following:

- Changes in body posture
- Grimacing
- Decreased willingness to participate in activities that would normally be engaging
- Somnolence due to exhaustion
- Increased nonspecific vocalization
- Agitation
- Crying
- Resistance to physical contact
- Resistance to ambulation

To successfully approach pain assessment and management in the cognitively impaired patient, the practitioner should realize that the most accurate data for assessing pain are obtained in the following order:

1. Patient's report of pain
2. Reports of patient's pain by family, friends, or other caregiver
3. Patient's behaviors
4. Physiologic parameters (most useful in acute pain)[26]

A possible recent event that is the cause of the pain (e.g., a recent fall) should be included in the investigation.

Clinicians should avoid relying on their own subjective judgment to estimate the degree of a patient's pain. Efforts should be directed toward seeing if a patient can use some form of self-report. The patient should be able to communicate the existence of pain through vocal or nonvocal communication and to rate the intensity of the pain. Several studies have demonstrated that elderly patients with mild to moderate cognitive impairment can respond fairly reliably to measures of pain intensity.[27-29]

The following steps recommended by the *Consensus Statement from the Veteran's Health Administration National Pain Management Strategy Coordinating Committee* are quite valuable in helping to try to assess and treat pain in the cognitively impaired patient:

■ **Observation of behaviors to assess pain**

■ When a patient is unable to use a self-report method despite efforts toward education, assessment must rely on observation of behaviors. Family members or consistent caregivers can provide valuable insight into the patient's usual behaviors and changes in behaviors that might indicate the presence of pain.[30]

■ Some common pain behaviors in cognitively impaired older persons have been identified.[30,31] These include signs mentioned previously. However, some patients with cognitive impairment exhibit little or no specific behaviors associated with pain. These pain behaviors have not been systematically evaluated in younger patients with cognitive impairments.

■ Pain behaviors should be observed and assessed both at rest and during movement.[28,32–34] Weiner and Herr[25] and others have noted that it is important to consider other causes of behaviors when relying on observation to assess pain. It is important to consider these other potential causes of distress behavior so that analgesic treatment does not mask problems, such as infections, constipation, bladder problems, and primary mood disorders.

■ **Empirical trials of analgesics**

■ Empirical trials of analgesic medication can be used as part of a pain assessment. This should be done in conjunction with other methods of assessment to evaluate the hypothesis that the behaviors are indicative of significant pain.[35, 36] This should not be a first-line method of assessment. There are no tested protocols for this practice. It is very important to consider other potential causes of distress behaviors or agitation that could be masked or worsened by analgesics. Many analgesics can negatively alter cognitive status, and this should be considered during the course of a trial. Changes in function and activity, as well as other pain behaviors, should always be assessed in the context of an analgesic trial.

■ **Tools for assessment of pain in cognitively impaired patients**

- A number of devices and protocols have been developed to aid in the assessment of patients who have impaired communication due to failures in cognition. These devices are based on observation of behaviors. Most of the available instruments have been developed for use with elderly patients. All the tools currently available suffer from a lack of studies to determine adequate reliability and validity. Clinicians should be very cautious about using an instrument that does not have established reliability and validity, even if it appears to have face value.[30]

A comprehensive review of currently published tools for assessing pain in nonverbal persons with dementia is available at The City of Hope Web site (www.cityofhope.org),[37] as listed below:

- Abbey Pain Scale[38]

- Assessment of Discomfort in Dementia[39]

- Checklist of Nonverbal Pain Indicators[40]

- Discomfort Scale-Dementia of the Alzheimer's Type[41]

- Doloplus 2[42]

- Face, Legs, Activity, Cry, and Consolability Pain Assessment Tool

- Nursing Assistant-Administered Instrument to Assess Pain in Demented Individuals[43]

- Pain Assessment in Advanced Dementia Scale[44]

- Pain Assessment for the Dementing Elderly[45]

- Pain Assessment Scale for Seniors with Severe Dementia[46]

Although successful treatment of pain in the cognitively impaired patient remains challenging, it is the clinician's responsibility to use all possible means available to successfully manage this difficult condition.

PATIENTS WITH SUBSTANCE ABUSE PROBLEMS

The risk of inadequately managing pain increases with patients with addictive disorders or substance abuse problems. It can be helpful to use objective screening and management tools, such as the **SOAPP**®[47] (**S**creener and **O**pioid **A**ssessment for **P**atients with **P**ain) and **COMM**™[48] (**C**urrent **O**pioid **M**isuse **M**easure), which can be downloaded from *www.PainEDU.org*.

Many factors are responsible for this undertreatment:

■ Inadequate clinician training in pain management and addiction medicine

■ Lack of acknowledged differences between dependence, addiction, and tolerance

■ Fear of contributing to addictive behavior by using opioids

■ Societal prejudices on patients with addictive disorders

■ Fear of regulatory penalization

Challenges in treating pain in this patient population are compounded by the patient's perception that the pain they experience is a major cause of their addictive behavior and also an obstacle to withdrawal of the offending agent. Patients with addictive disorders sometimes have problems managing opioids by themselves, and this may indeed lead them to be deprived of a potentially valuable component of their pain treatment.

In 2001, 21 health organizations and the Drug Enforcement Administration released *"Promoting Pain Relief and Preventing Abuse of Pain Medications: A Critical Balancing Act,"* which states the following important points with respect to pain management in patients with substance abuse problems[49]:

> "As representatives of the health care community and law enforcement, we are working together to prevent abuse of prescription pain medications while ensuring that they remain available for patients in need.

Both health care professionals, and law enforcement and regulatory personnel, share a responsibility for ensuring that prescription pain medications are available to the patients who need them and for preventing these drugs from becoming a source of harm or abuse. We all must ensure that accurate information about both the legitimate use and the abuse of prescription pain medications is made available. The roles of both health professionals and law enforcement personnel in maintaining this essential balance between patient care and diversion prevention are critical.

Preventing drug abuse is an important societal goal, but there is consensus, by law enforcement agencies, health care practitioners, and patient advocates alike, that it should not hinder patients' ability to receive the care they need and deserve."

This consensus statement is based on the following facts:

- Undertreatment of pain is a serious problem in the United States, including pain among patients with chronic conditions and those who are critically ill or near death. Effective pain management is an integral and important aspect of quality medical care, and pain should be treated aggressively.

- For many patients, opioid analgesics, when used as recommended by established pain management guidelines, are the most effective way to treat their pain and often the only treatment option that provides significant relief.

- Because opioids are one of several types of controlled substances that have potential for abuse, they are carefully regulated by the Drug Enforcement Administration and other state agencies. For example, a clinician must be licensed by state medical authorities and registered with the Drug Enforcement Administration before prescribing a controlled substance.

- In spite of regulatory controls, drug abusers obtain these and other prescription medications by diverting them from legitimate channels in several ways, including fraud, theft, forged prescriptions, and via unscrupulous health professionals.

- Drug abuse is a serious problem. Those who legally manufacture, distribute, prescribe, and dispense controlled substances must be mindful of and have respect for their inherent abuse potential. Focusing only on the abuse potential of a drug, however, could erroneously lead to the conclusion that these medications should be avoided when medically indicated, generating a sense of fear rather than respect for their legitimate properties.

- Helping doctors, nurses, pharmacists, other health care professionals, law enforcement personnel, and the general public to become more aware of both the use and abuse of pain medications enables all clinicians to make proper and wise decisions regarding the treatment of pain.

Below is a table with some basic principles and strategies for using opioids in the patient with a known substance abuse problem. Never forget that consultation with a specialist in pain management may always be a valuable choice in management of difficult patient populations.

■ Table 7.4
Strategies of Opioid Use in the Patient with Known History of Substance Abuse

- **Support the individual** to help achieve and sustain recovery from addiction.
- **Provide medications in manageable amounts** to patients.
- **Use schedules and dosages that are less likely to cause euphoric effects,** but retain efficacy.
- **Require a written agreement** between you and the patient with respect to abuse of prescribed medications.
- **Communicate as appropriately necessary with significant others.**
- **See patients frequently** to assess for signs and symptoms of abuse.
- If there are signs of medication abuse, **obtain frequent urine screens, schedule frequent clinic visits, and encourage substance abuse counseling.**
- **If safety concerns outweigh the potential of treatment, discontinue opioid therapy,** and use nonopioid approaches.

REFERENCES

1. Krechel SW, Bildner J. CRIES: a new neonatal postoperative pain measurement score. Initial testing of validity and reliability. *Paediatr Anaesth.* 1995;5(1):53–61.

2. Merkel SI, Shayefitz JR, Lewis TV, Malwiya S. The FLACC: a behavioral scale for scoring postoperative pain in young children. *Pediatr Nurs.* 1997;23(3):293–297.

3. Jacox AK, Carr DB, Payne R, et al. Management of Cancer Pain, Clinical Practice Guidelines. No. 9. Rockville, MD: U.S. Department of Health and Human Services, Public Health Service, Agency for Health Care Policy and Research (AHCPR Publication No. 94-0592), 1994.

4. Sorkin BA, Rudy TE, Hanlon RB, Turk DC. Chronic pain in older and young patients: differences appear less important than similarities. *J Gerontol.* 1990;45(2):64–68.

5. American Geriatrics Society Panel on Pharmacological Management of Persistent Pain in Older Persons. Pharmacological management of persistent pain in older persons. *J Am Geriatr Soc.* 2009 Aug;57(8):1331–1346. Epub 2009 Jul 2.

6. American Geriatrics Society Panel on Pharmacological Management of Persistent Pain in Older Persons. Pharmacological management of persistent pain in older persons (executive summary). 2009. http://www.americangeriatrics.org/health_care_professionals/clinical_practice/clinical_guidelines_recommendations/persistent_pain_executive_summary. Accessed July 8, 2010.

7. United States Food and Drug Administration. Current Categories for Drug Use in Pregnancy. Federal Register 1980;44:37434–67.

8. U.S. Census Bureau. An older and more diverse nation by midcentury [press release]. 2008 Aug 14. http://www.census.gov/newsroom/releases/archives/population/cb08-123.html. Accessed July 8, 2010.

9. National Cancer Institute. Center to Reduce Cancer Health Disparities. Health disparities defined. http://crchd.cancer.gov/disparities/defined.html. Updated August 24, 2009. Accessed July 7, 2010.

10. Todd KH, Samaroo N, Hoffman JR. Ethnicity as a risk factor for inadequate emergency department analgesia. *JAMA.* 1993 Mar 24-31;269(12):1537–1539.

11. Morrison RS, Wallenstein S, Natale DK, Senzel RS, Huang LL. "We don't carry that"--failure of pharmacies in predominantly nonwhite neighborhoods to stock opioid analgesics. *N Engl J Med.* 2000 Apr 6;342(14):1023–1026.

12. Green CR, Ndao-Brumblay SK, West B, Washington T. Differences in prescription opioid analgesic availability: comparing minority and white pharmacies across Michigan. *J Pain*. 2005 Oct;6(10):689–699.

13. Smedley BD, Stith AY, Nelson AR, eds. *Unequal Treatment: Confronting Racial and Ethnic Disparities in Healthcare*. Washington, DC: National Academies Press; 2003.

14. U.S. Department of Health and Human Services. *Healthy People 2010: Understanding and Improving Health*. 2nd ed. Washington, DC: U.S. Government Printing Office; November 2000.

15. Anderson KO, Green CR, Payne R. Racial and ethnic disparities in pain: causes and consequences of unequal care. *J Pain*. 2009 Dec;10(12):1187–1204.

16. Morris DB. Sociocultural dimensions of pain management. In: Fishman SM, Ballantyne JC, Rathmell JP, eds. *Bonica's Management of Pain*. 4th ed. Philadelphia: Lippincott Williams & Wilkins; 2009:133–145.

17. Veterans Health Administration. VHA National Pain Management Strategy. Washington (DC): Department of Veterans Affairs; 1998.

18. Veterans Health Administration. VHA Directive 2009–053: Pain management. Washington (DC): Department of Veterans Affairs; 2009. http://www1.va.gov/PAINMANAGEMENT/docs/VHA09PainDirective.pdf. Accessed July 7, 2010.

19. Veterans Health Administration. VHA National Pain Management Strategy Teleconference Call. 2009.

20. Lew HL, Otis JD, Tun C, Kerns RD, Clark ME, Cifu DX. Prevalence of chronic pain, posttraumatic stress disorder, and persistent postconcussive symptoms in OIF/OEF veterans: polytrauma clinical triad. *J Rehabil Res Dev*. 2009;46(6):697–702.

21. Tanielian T, Jaycox LH, eds. *Invisible Wounds of War: Psychological and Cognitive Injuries, Their Consequences, and Services to Assist Recovery*. Santa Monica, CA: Rand Corporation; 2008.

22. Centers for Medicare and Medicaid Services. *Medicare Hospice Benefits*. Washington (DC): U.S. Department of Health and Human Services, Health Care Financing Administration; 2010. http://www.medicare.gov/publications/pubs/pdf/02154.pdf. Accessed July 7, 2010.

23. National Consensus Project for Quality Palliative Care. *Clinical Practice Guidelines for Quality Palliative Care*. 2nd ed. Pittsburgh (PA): National Consensus Project for Quality Palliative Care; 2009.

24. Paice JA. Pain management at the end of life. In: Fishman SM, Ballantyne JC, Rathmell JP, eds. *Bonica's Management of Pain*. 4th ed. Philadelphia: Lippincott Williams & Wilkins;2009:1547–1557.

25. Weiner DK, Herr K. Comprehensive interdisciplinary assessment and treatment planning: an integrated overview. In: Weiner DK, Herr K, Rudy TE, eds. *Persistent Pain in Older Adults: An Interdisciplinary Guide for Treatment*. New York: Springer Publishing Company; 2002:18–57.

26. Assessing Pain in the Patient with Impaired Communication: A Consensus Statement from the VHA National Pain Management Strategy Coordinating Committee. 2004. http://www1.va.gov/PAINMANAGEMENT/docs/Cognitivelyimpairedconsensusstatement.doc. Accessed July 7, 2010.

27. Chibnall J, Tait R. Pain assessment in cognitively impaired and unimpaired older adults: a comparison of four scales. *Pain*. 2001;92:173–186.

28. Weiner MF, Koss E, Patterson M, et al. A comparison of the Cohen-Mansfield agitation inventory with the CERAD behavioral rating scale for dementia in community-dwelling persons with Alzheimer's disease. *J Psychiatr Res*. 1998 Nov-Dec;32(6):347–351.

29. Ferrell BA, Ferrell BR, Rivera L. Pain in cognitively impaired nursing home patients. *J Pain Symptom Manage*. 1995;10(8):591–598.

30. Herr K, Garand L, American Geriatric Society Panel on Persistent Pain in Older Persons. The management of persistent pain in older persons. *J Am Geriatr Soc*. 2001;50:S205–S224.

31. Asplund K, Norberg A, Adolfsson R, Waxman HM. Facial expressions in severely demented patients: a stimulus-response study of four patients with dementia of the Alzheimer's type. *Int J Geriatr Psychiatry*. 1991;6:599–606.

32. Feldt KS. The checklist of nonverbal pain indicators. *Pain Manag Nurs*. 2000;1:13–21.

33. Feldt KS, Ryden M, Miles S. Treatment of pain in cognitively impaired compared with cognitively intact older patients with hip fractures. *J Am Geriatr Soc*. 1998;46(9):1079–1085.

34. Weiner D, Pieper C, McConnell E, et al. Pain measurement in elders with chronic low back pain: traditional and alternative approaches. *Pain*. 1996;67(2–3):461–467.

35. Baker A, Bowring L, Brignell A, Kafford D. Chronic pain management in cognitively impaired patients: a preliminary research project. *Perspectives*. 1996;20(2):4–8.

36. Kovach CR, Weissman DE, Griffie J, et al. Assessment and treatment of discomfort for people with late-stage dementia. *J Pain Symptom Manage*. 1999;18:412–419.

37. City of Hope Pain & Palliative Care Resource Center. Pain Resource Center: Pain in the Elderly. http://prc.coh.org/elderly.asp. Accessed July 8, 2010.

38. Abbey J, Piller N, De Bellis A, et al. The Abbey Pain Scale: a 1-minute numerical indicator for people with end-stage dementia. *Int J Palliat Nurs*. 2004;10(1):6–13.

39. Kovach CR, Weissman DE, Griffie J, et al. Assessment and treatment of discomfort for people with late-stage dementia. *J Pain Symptom Manage*. 1999;18:412–419.

40. Feldt KS. The checklist of nonverbal pain indicators. *Pain Manag Nurs*. 2000;1:13–21.

41. Hurley AC, Volicer B, Hanrahan PA, et al. Assessment of discomfort in advanced Alzheimer patients. *Res Nurs Health*. 1992;15(5):369–377.

42. Wary B. Doloplus-2, une echelle pour evaluer la douleur. *Soins Gerontol*. 1999;19:25–27.

43. Snow AL, O'Malley K, Kunik M, et al. A conceptual model of pain assessment for non-communicative persons with dementia. *Gerontologist*. 2004;44:807–817.

44. Warden V, Hurley AC, Volicer L. Development and psychometric evaluation of the Pain Assessment in Advanced Dementia (PAINAD) scale. *J Am Med Dir Assoc*. 2003 Jan-Feb;4(1):9-15.

45. Villanueva MR, Smith TL, Erickson JS, Lee AC, Singer CM. Pain Assessment for the Dementing Elderly (PADE): reliability and validity of a new measure. *J Am Med Dir Assoc*. 2003 Jan-Feb;4(1):1–8.

46. Zwakhalen SM, Hamers JP, Berger MP. Improving the clinical usefulness of a behavioural pain scale for older people with dementia. *J Adv Nurs*. 2007 Jun;58(5):493–502. Epub 2007 Apr 17.

47. Butler SF, Budman SH, Fernandez K, et al. Validation of a screener and opioid assessment measure for patients with chronic pain. *Pain*. 2004;112:65–75.

48. Butler SF, Budman, SH, Fernandez K, et al. Development and validation of the Current Opioid Misuse Measure. *Pain*. 2007;130:144–156.

49. Drug Enforcement Administration. A joint statement from 21 health organizations and the Drug Enforcement Administration. Promoting pain relief and preventing abuse of pain medications: a critical balancing act. *J Pain Symptom Manage*. 2002 Aug;24(2):147.

VIII.

Patient Level Opioid Risk Management

RISKS OF OPIOID THERAPY

As chronic pain continues to be a major public health problem in the United States, its incidence is steadily rising. Improved diagnostic methods, ongoing research, the baby boomers increasing in age, and increased emphasis on thorough pain assessment are some of the reasons responsible for this escalation. As opioids remain an essential tool, in many cases as part of the armamentarium for the treatment of chronic pain unresponsive to other interventions, it stands to reason that the frequency of their use increases in parallel with the incidence of chronic pain. Additionally, owing to substantial efforts to improve awareness and treatment of chronic pain, the availability of opioids has increased dramatically in the past several decades. Although much more remains to be done to ensure appropriate access to opioids, opioid prescribing is currently at the highest level ever, allowing patients with cancer and noncancer pain unprecedented access to these analgesics.

As with all medications, prescription of opioids is associated with certain risks, and the prevalence of negative consequences of opioid use has risen concomitantly with their increased use by health care providers. In many cases, these risks are similar to that of other medications, and in other cases they are different. Although addiction gets significant media attention, other things also need to be taken into consideration by clinicians about the appropriate role of opioid analgesia and associated risks. Common risks of opioid therapy include adverse effects, drug interactions, consumption with alcohol, diversion, and aberrant drug-related behaviors.

Adverse Effects

The development of adverse effects from opioids should always guide clinicians to weigh the treatment risks against the expected benefits. Anticipating potential adverse effects in relation to predisposing patient factors can be critical when addressing this problem. The mechanisms by which opioids cause these adverse effects are not always completely understood, and can vary from patient to patient. For example, gender, race, genetics, and increasing age are all factors that have been shown to influence the development of adverse effects. Additionally, physiologic compromise, such as reduction in renal or hepatic function, and other comorbid conditions may lead to accumulation of opioids and their metabolites, increasing the likelihood of adverse effects. Few randomized comparative studies have evaluated the safety and effectiveness of various treatment regimens to manage adverse effects of opioids. Many of the recommendations for management are based on consensus opinion and clinical experience.[1]

Some basic approaches to management of adverse effects include:

- **Dose reduction**
- **Symptomatic management**
- **Opioid rotation**
- **Alternative route of administration**

Chapter VI discusses management of specific opioid-related adverse effects.

Drug Interactions

Many patients with chronic pain have comorbid medical conditions requiring medical treatment that may complicate opioid therapy. Additionally, selecting the appropriate opioid not only requires knowledge of *how* individual opioids differ with respect to metabolism and interaction with concurrent medications, but also reasons *why* specific medical conditions may influence their efficacy and tolerability.[2]

Polypharmacy is a common complicating condition in the elderly and in patients with psychiatric illness, cancer, cardiovascular disease, diabetes mellitus or other chronic illnesses, which can increase the risk of drug interactions in these patient populations. *Pharmacokinetic interactions* can alter exposure to the opioid or concurrent medications, thereby potentially reducing efficacy and/or tolerability, and possibly increasing the likelihood of adverse effects or even toxicity. *Pharmacodynamic interactions* can enhance the depressive effects of opioids, compromising safety, especially in patients with impaired renal or hepatic function, who may have difficulty clearing or metabolizing opioids and concurrent medications, leading to increased risk of adverse events. Patients with cardiovascular, cerebrovascular, or respiratory disease may require a higher level of vigilance for respiratory depression, bradycardia, and hypotension, which could occur with any opioid. Patients with cerebrovascular disease, dementia, brain injury, or psychiatric illness are also more susceptible to opioid effects on the CNS, which can include euphoria, cognitive impairment, and sedation. In addition to prescription medication polypharmacy, *it is also important to consider the interaction of other substances* with opioids, such as illicit drugs, over-the-counter medications, certain foods, and herbal substances. Appropriate opioid selection along with a detailed history could help to mitigate these effects and positively influence clinical judgment with respect to the risk/benefit analysis.

Consumption with Alcohol

Opioids may also interact with alcohol resulting in undesirable outcomes. As with polypharmacy, there are generally two types of alcohol drug interactions: *pharmacokinetic* and *pharmacodynamic*. Pharmacokinetic interactions occur when alcohol alters the metabolism or excretion of the drug or vice versa. Pharmacodynamic interactions refer to the *additive effects* of alcohol and certain drugs, particularly in the central nervous system (e.g., sedation) without affecting the pharmacokinetics of the drug.[3] Alcohol is primarily metabolized in the liver by several enzymes. The most important enzymes are aldehyde dehydrogenase and CYP2E1. In people who consume alcohol only occasionally,

CYP2E1 metabolizes only a small fraction of the ingested alcohol. In contrast, chronic heavy drinking can increase CYP2E1 activity up to tenfold, resulting in a higher proportion of alcohol being metabolized by CYP2E1, rather than aldehyde dehydrogenase. Therefore, in some cases, the effect of alcohol on the interacting drug may be different depending on chronic or acute alcohol use.[4,5]

The following list contains examples of possible consequences of interaction of opioids with consumed alcohol:

- **Tolerance**
- **Increased release rate and absorption**, which may lead to unexpected potentially fatal doses
- **Interactions with extended-release mechanisms**, resulting in a "dumping effect"
- **Impaired psychomotor performance**
- **Enhanced CNS depression**, potentially resulting in obtundation, respiratory depression, hypotension, coma, or in some cases, death

Diversion

Diversion of prescribed opioid medications has received a lot of media attention, and is considered to be many different things to different people. Broadly defined, diversion is when the legal supply chain of prescription medications is circumvented, and drugs are transferred from a licit to an illicit channel of distribution or use. Concern exists regarding the increasing rates of diversion correlating to the increasing rates of prescriptions written. The challenge lies in maintaining the legal distribution to patients in need while stemming the tide of diversion. Often, opioid-related deaths resulting from misuse or diversion receive intense media attention. Blame is often directed towards prescribers, exacerbating fears about medical use of prescription drugs among both patients and providers. This increases concerns about regulatory scrutiny.

It is accurate to say that the opportunity for diversion exists at almost every step in the process, from the manufacturing and distribution side to the prescription and patient side, and everywhere in between. When controlled substances are lost or stolen along the manufacturing and supply chain, pharmacists, manufacturers, and distributors must report these occurrences to the U.S. Drug Enforcement Administration. DEA data reveal that in the 4-year period from 2000 through 2003, nearly 28 million dosage units of all controlled substances were diverted by theft or loss from lawful channels, of which 24% were opioid analgesics.[6]

A unique feature of prescription drug abuse complicating medical prescribing is that problems may occur not only in patients, but also in their family and friends. Since prescribed opioids can be a major source of abused substances for others, it is clear that at times the patients receiving valid prescriptions can actually *become* the source of these medications that put the community at risk. This pathway of diversion may be intentional (the patient knows that giving or selling is wrong), unintentional (the patient thinks they can help by giving medication), or by theft (e.g., stolen from the patient's medicine cabinet or purse). Prescribers therefore, have unique obligations to prescribe opioids in a manner that minimizes potential harm to *non-patients*, as well as patients.

The societal implications of opioid diversion are extremely important, and should be addressed at both a clinical and law enforcement level. Clinicians and regulatory agencies must employ efforts to prevent drug diversion that are evidence-based, not media-driven, and that do not result in the inadequate treatment of pain patients in need.

Aberrant Drug-Related Behaviors

Often the prescription opioid-related risks of greatest concern have been aberrant drug-related behaviors, including misuse, abuse, and addiction. An important step in the process of understanding aberrant drug-related behaviors and their risks involves comprehension of the terminology[7]:

- **Misuse**   Use of a medication (*for a medical purpose*) other than as directed or as indicated, whether willful or unintentional, and whether harm results or not

- **Abuse**   *Any* use of a legal or illegal medication or substance by intentional self-administration *for a nonmedical purpose*, such as altering one's state of consciousness (e.g., "getting high")

■ *Physical dependence*　The state of adaptation that is manifested by a drug class-specific withdrawal syndrome that can be produced by abrupt cessation, rapid dose reduction, decreasing blood level of the drug, and administration of an antagonist

■ *Tolerance*　The state of adaptation in which exposure to a given dose of a drug induces biologic changes that result in diminution of one or more of the drug's effects over time. Alternatively, escalating doses of a drug are required over time to maintain a given level of effect

■ *Addiction*　A primary, chronic neurobiologic disease with genetic, psychosocial, and environmental factors influencing its development and manifestations. Behavioral characteristics include one or more of the following:

　■ Impaired control over drug use

　■ Compulsive use

　■ Continued use despite harm

　■ Craving

■ *Iatrogenic*　Denoting response to medical or surgical treatment induced by treatment itself (*usually used for unfavorable responses*)

■ *Pseudoaddiction*　Syndrome of abnormal behavior resulting from undertreatment of pain that is misidentified by the clinician as inappropriate drug-seeking behavior

　■ Behavior ceases when adequate pain relief is provided

　■ Not a diagnosis; rather, a description of a clinical interaction

■ *Diversion*　The intentional removal of a medication from legitimate distribution and dispensing channels

Some data suggest that prescription opioid abuse is rising faster than any other type of drug abuse and is now second only to marijuana in terms of prevalence of abuse and addiction, and ahead of cocaine and heroin by many measures. Even among older Americans (50 and older), where new substance abuse admissions data show sharp increases in the proportion being treated for illicit substances such as cocaine, heroin, and marijuana, prescription drug abuse is a significant problem. A recent SAMHSA study report showed that from 1992 to 2008 the proportion of admissions among this age group due primarily to prescription drug abuse rose, from 0.7 percent to 3.5 percent.[8] Additionally, in 2008, cocaine abuse was the leading primary cause of admissions involving substances initiated in the past five years among older Americans (26.2 percent), with prescription drug misuse a close second (25.8 percent).

Current projections suggest that approximately 1.5 million Americans meet criteria for abuse or addiction to prescription opioids, which is about 0.5% of the population. There may be significant overlap between patients with pain and those with addictive disorders, so it is likely that no clinician is free from treating patients with comorbid pain and addiction. This becomes clear when one considers that the background rate of active substance abuse is approximately somewhere between 3.8–10% in the general U.S. population[9] and the fact that pain is one of the most common reasons for patients to seek medical attention. The presence of comorbid addiction significantly complicates the treatment of pain, and the presence of comorbid pain significantly complicates the treatment of addiction.

REGULATION OF OPIOIDS

The use of opioid analgesics in the United States is governed by a combination of regulatory policies at federal and state levels.

At the state level, responsible prescribing of opioids is encouraged by guidelines developed by the Federation of the State Medical Boards of the United States (FSMB)[10] whose mission is to "continuously improve the quality, safety, and integrity of health care through developing and promoting high standards for physician licensure and practice."

Opioid analgesics are also subject to laws governed by the Controlled Substances Act of 1970 and enforced by the Drug Enforcement Administration (DEA). The Controlled Substances Act (CSA)[11] requires that certain drugs be placed in one of five *controlled substance schedules*, based upon medical value, safety and potential for abuse or addiction:

■ **Schedule I**

- Drugs or other substances that have *no currently accepted* (in the United States) *medicinal value*; lack of, or poor demonstration of safety; and a *high potential for abuse*. Examples are substances such as heroin, lysergic acid diethylamide (LSD), marijuana, and methaqualone.

■ **Schedule II**

- Drugs or other substances that *currently have an accepted medical use* (in the United States), have a *high potential for abuse, and may lead to psychological and/or physical dependence*. Examples are commonly used opioid analgesics, such as oxycodone, morphine, fentanyl, and hydromorphone.

■ **Schedule III**

- Drugs or other substances that have a *currently accepted medical use (in the United States), have a lower potential of abuse than that of schedule I or II drugs or substances, and whose abuse may lead to a moderate or low level of psychological and/or physical dependence*. Examples are substances such as anabolic steroids, hydrocodone with aspirin or acetaminophen, and codeine.

■ **Schedule IV**

- Drugs or other substances that have a currently accepted medical use (in the United States), have a *low potential for abuse relative to schedule III drugs or other substances, and whose abuse may lead to limited psychological and/or physical dependence relative to schedule III drugs*. Examples are substances such as benzodiazepines, partial agonist opioid analgesics, such as pentazocine and propoxyphene.

■ **Schedule V**

- Drugs or other substances that have a currently accepted medical use (in the United States), have a *low potential for abuse* relative to schedule IV drugs or other substances, and whose abuse may lead to limited psychological and/or physical dependence relative to schedule IV drugs. Examples are substances such as cough suppressants with small amounts of codeine, and pregabalin.

RiskMAPs and REMS

The *Food and Drug Administration (FDA)* is charged with approval to market medications that are deemed as safe and effective for medical use. Once approved by the FDA, a drug may be prescribed as labeled, or in an "off-label" manner, at the prescribing clinician's discretion based on a therapeutic risk/benefit evaluation and conformity to community standards of good medical practice.

In 2002, Congress reauthorized, for the third time, the *Prescription Drug User Fee Act (PDUFA III)*. One of the goals of *PDUFA* was to produce guidance for the pharmaceutical industry on risk management activities for drug and biological products. The intent of the FDA was to create a plan that would encompass the idea of ***medication risk management***.

Specifically, medication risk management is described by the FDA as an iterative four-part process that should be continuous throughout a medication's life cycle, with the results of risk assessment informing the manufacturer's further decisions regarding risk minimization:

1. Assessing a medication's risk-benefit balance

2. Developing and implementing tools to minimize risks while preserving benefits

3. Evaluating tool effectiveness and reassessing the risk-benefit balance

4. Making adjustments, as appropriate, to the risk minimization tools to further improve the risk-benefit balance

Within the context of medication risk management, part of the application to the FDA for approval may require submission by the manufacturer of a ***Risk Minimization Action Plan or RiskMAP***. The FDA defines a *RiskMAP* as the *"strategic safety program designed to meet specific goals and objectives in minimizing known risks of a medication while preserving its benefits."* For the majority of FDA-approved products, labeling and routine reporting requirements of adverse events are sufficient to mitigate risks and preserve benefits. In a relatively small number of cases, when additional measures are deemed necessary to ensure that the benefits of a drug outweigh the risks, a *RiskMAP* is required. The intent of a submitted *RiskMAP* is to lay out a plan (processes or systems) to minimize known safety risks, including risks of adverse effects, aberrant drug-related behaviors, and negative outcomes relative to the risk. The submitted plan is to include processes such as:

1. Targeted education and outreach to health care practitioners or patients to communicate risks and appropriate safety behaviors

2. Reminder systems, processes, or forms to foster reduced-risk prescribing and use

3. Performance-linked access systems that guide prescribing, dispensing, and use of the product to target the population and conditions of use most likely to confer benefits and to minimize particular risks

Decisions by the FDA to require a RiskMAP are made based on the Agency's own interpretation of risk information, on a case-by-case basis, and continue today.

In September 2007, the President signed into law H.R. 3580, the **Food and Drug Administration Amendments Act of 2007 (FDAAA)**. This new law represented a **significant addition to FDA authority**.

Among the many components of the FDAAA law, the PDUFA, which was nearing expiration, was reauthorized and expanded. The resulting law contained numerous provisions designed to:

- Better inform the public about drug safety
- Provide new tools for the FDA to reduce risks and unsafe drug use

The passage of the FDAAA:

- Enhanced the FDA's authority to require drug labeling changes and additional post-market studies
- Gave the FDA the authority to require **Risk Evaluation and Mitigation Strategies (REMS)** for new products and already approved products, if it becomes aware of new safety information

and determines that a *REMS* is necessary to "ensure the benefits of the drug outweigh the risks of the drug".

- *REMS* expanded assessment of medication risk management, previously built into *RiskMAPs*, to include periodic reassessment and modification as necessary.

- Contents of *REMS* include:
  - A Medication Guide
  - A patient package insert, if such insert may help mitigate a serious risk of the drug
  - Elements to assure safe use of the medication
  - A communication plan to convey to health care providers information that supports the mitigation strategy

- Granted the FDA the authority to require additional post-approval studies; and, if marketed medications are found to be associated with new potential risks, the FDA can require labeling changes or additional research to address these risks

- Stopped the FDA short of requiring *REMS* for all new drugs, as was originally proposed; the FDA would therefore decide on a case-by-case basis whether a drug that is pending approval warrants a *REMS*

Manufacturers that fail to make FDA-requested labeling changes or to conduct timely post-market studies would be found to be in violation of the FDAAA, and subject to fines. Pharmaceutical companies could also be penalized for failing to implement a requested, submitted, and approved *REMS*.

The FDAAA, *REMS*, and pain management with chronic opioid therapy crossed paths in early 2009,[12] when the FDA sent letters to manufacturers of all extended-release opioid drugs, indicating that these drugs will be required to have a *REMS* in addition to their *RiskMAPs* to ensure that the benefits of the drugs continue to outweigh the risks of:

1. Use of certain opioid products in non-opioid-tolerant individuals

2. Abuse

3. Overdose, both *accidental* and *intentional*

The FDA stated in this letter that:

- "The agency has long been concerned about adverse events associated with this class of drug and has taken steps in cooperation with drug manufacturers to address these risks. We intend to use the agency's *REMS* authority under the Food and Drug Administration Amendments Act of 2007 (FDAAA) to mitigate the risks of these drugs."

- "Opioid drugs have benefit when used properly and are a necessary component of pain management for certain patients."

- "Opioid drugs have serious risks when used improperly."

- "The FDA, drug manufacturers, and others have taken a number of steps in the past to prevent misuse, abuse and accidental overdose of these drugs, including providing additional warnings in product labeling, implementing risk management plans (*RiskMAPs*), conducting inter-agency collaborations, and issuing direct communications to both prescribers and patients."

  - "Despite these efforts, the rates of misuse and abuse, and of accidental overdose of opioids, have risen over the past decade."

- "The FDA believes that establishing a *REMS* for opioids will reduce these risks, while still ensuring that patients with legitimate need for these drugs will continue to have appropriate access."

- "The *REMS* would be intended to ensure that the benefits of these drugs continue to outweigh certain risks."

All companies that make extended-release opioids have been asked by the FDA to work together, as opposed to separately, to create a single, broad-application *REMS* program that will encompass all extended-release medications in this class. Although individual medications have been required the submission of a *REMS* as part of their application, or to implement one post-FDA approval, this is the first time that the FDA has indicated that a *REMS* will be needed on a class-wide basis. The likely impetus is the number of drug-related deaths associated with extended-release opioids.

Once a clear direction exists, the FDA will likely consult with the DEA on the class-wide *REMS*. The Controlled Substances Act and DEA regulations that require manufacturers and registrants of controlled substances to maintain effective controls against diversion and compliance with *REMS*, could arguably be viewed as a part of this duty. Drug manufacturers will need to consider that the DEA will evaluate compliance with *REMS* as a factor in determining ongoing compliance with DEA requirements.

Clinical Implications

The *REMS* for extended-release opioids needs to provide mechanisms that will likely include a variety of elements to assure safe use of these medications, and to ensure that *prescribers, dispensers, and patients* are all aware of, and understand, the risks and appropriate use of these products.

There is little doubt that the finalized program will likely have requirements that have some degree of clinical impact at all stakeholder levels:

- Ongoing, opioid-specific training and possibly certification for clinicians and pharmacists

- A higher level of clinician vigilance than previously required

- Expanded use of doctor-patient opioid agreements
  - Detailing the responsibilities of both clinician and patient
  - Including review and confirmation of patient comprehension of the Medication Guide for the specific medication
  - Including dissemination of information about the safe and appropriate use of opioid medications, and the dangers of sharing medications

- A plan that outlines continued monitoring of these initiatives to ensure that the goals are being met

The challenge will be to ensure access to patients in need that are appropriate candidates for extended-release opioids, while achieving the desired goals.

State Policies and Regulations

All clinicians must be familiar with the rules regarding controlled-substance prescribing in their states. Such regulations control activities such as calling in prescriptions, writing refills, calling in emergency supplies, and so forth. Prescribing opioids to patients with pain in the course of usual medical practice, and in the context of a legitimate doctor–patient relationship, is permitted. Moreover, the courts increasingly expect clinicians to attend to patients' pain issues, including if the use of opioid analgesics is required. It is rare for physicians acting in the context of appropriate medical practice, and maintaining adequate records, to be censured for prescribing opioids to patients with pain.

One common source of confusion is whether physicians can prescribe to patients with addiction. The simple answer is that physicians with current licenses and DEA registrations can indeed prescribe opioids, including methadone and buprenorphine, to patients with pain, whether or not the patient has an addictive disorder (although this may not always be advisable). To prescribe for the "maintenance treatment" of addiction, a physician must have a special license or waiver, whether or not the patient has pain. Of course, in the patient with comorbid pain and addiction, it may not be clear under which regulation the medication is prescribed to treat pain or the addiction. Nonetheless, physicians must be mindful of the applicable regulations. Unless specially licensed, physicians must be prescribing for pain, not addiction, even in patients with comorbid addictive disorders, and the medical chart must reflect this practice.

OPIOID RISK MINIMIZATION IN CLINICAL PRACTICE

"Clinical Guidelines for the Use of Chronic Opioid Therapy in Chronic Noncancer Pain"

The American Pain Society (APS), in partnership with the American Academy of Pain Medicine (AAPM), commissioned a multidisciplinary panel of 21 experts that worked for over a year to develop evidence-based guidelines on chronic opioid therapy in adults with noncancer pain.[13]

The rationale for developing these guidelines was based on the impression that "Risk stratification pertaining to outcomes associated with the abuse liability of opioids—misuse, abuse, addiction and diversion—is a vital but relatively undeveloped skill for many clinicians. However, all clinicians prescribing opioids should be knowledgeable about risk factors for opioid abuse and methods for assessing risk. Clinicians should also assess for opioid-associated adverse effects, given their high prevalence."[13]

These guidelines, published in February 2009, are based on a comprehensive and systematic review of published evidence on the subject. The guidelines are slated to be reviewed and updated by 2012. Importantly, these guidelines are targeted towards both *primary care and specialty settings*, essentially "all clinicians who provide care for adults with chronic noncancer pain, including cancer survivors with chronic pain due to their cancer or its treatment."

The following summarizes the key 14 recommendations:

1. **Patient Selection and Risk Stratification**

   Proper patient selection is paramount in the process of opioid therapy, including weighing the specific benefits and risks of treatment, and completing a thorough risk assessment.

   a. *Prior* to initiating chronic opioid therapy

   i. **A detailed history and physical** is necessary as well as assessment **of risk** of likelihood of abuse, misuse, or addiction (***Proper patient selection*** *is critical and requires a comprehensive benefit-to-harm evaluation that weighs the potential positive effects of opioids on pain and function against potential risks. **Thorough risk assessment and stratification is appropriate in every case.***)

   ii. **Clinicians may consider a trial of chronic opioid therapy** if the pain is moderate or severe, if the pain has a significant impact on quality of life, and if potential benefits outweigh potential risks.

iii. **Documentation** of a "benefit-to-harm" evaluation should be performed before, and on an ongoing basis throughout the course of therapy.

2. Informed Consent and Opioid Management Plans

Patients need to be informed of the determined risks and benefits of treatment before initiating what should be considered a trial of therapy. Patients also need to be informed about the plan for management, and should understand the components of the plan.

a. **Informed consent** for opioid therapy should include items that any informed consent should contain:

i. Goals of treatment

ii. Expectations of treatment

iii. Risks and alternatives

b. **A written opioid management plan** should be considered (**www.PainEDU.org** has more information about opioid agreements, including sample agreements)

In patients already on chronic opioid therapy, "clinicians should periodically review risks and benefits of therapy. Patients should be counseled about the **potential for common opioid-related adverse effects** (e.g., constipation, nausea, sedation) as well as other serious risks" (e.g.,abuse, addiction, overdose). Potential **risks of long-term use or high-dose should also be discussed**.

3. Initiation and Titration of Chronic Opioid Therapy

Outcomes of opioid therapy that are important to consider include progress towards identified treatment goals, presence of medication-related side-effects, changes in the underlying source of the pain, and the identification of aberrant drug-related behaviors.

a. **Initial treatment should *always*** be considered **as a trial of therapy,** and be considered individually determined—not a definitive course of treatment.

b. Opioid selection, dosing, and titration should be tailored towards the patient's health status, previous opioid experience, goals of treatment, and identified or predicted possible harms of opioid therapy. "In patients who are opioid-naive, or have modest previous opioid exposure, opioids should be started at a low dose and titrated slowly, to decrease risk of opioid-related adverse effects°. In general, opioid doses should be individualized based on risk of adverse outcomes and responses to therapy. Some patients, such as frail older persons or those with comorbidities, may benefit from more cautious initiation and titration of therapy."

4. Use of Methadone

Methadone should be started at low doses and titrated slowly, in both opioid-experienced and opioid-tolerant patients.

a. Because of its complicated and variable pharmacokinetics and pharmacodynamics, the use of methadone is **recommended to be utilized only by clinicians familiar with its use and risks**.

b. Because of its long half-life and variable pharmacokinetics, the panel recommends that methadone **not be used to treat breakthrough pain** or as an as-needed medication.

5. Monitoring Patients

All patients on chronic opioid therapy should be periodically reassessed. The critical nature of this step is based on the fact that pain conditions frequently can change, and patients may develop new underlying conditions that could affect the treatment plan. The approach to monitoring is often guided by the assessment and risk stratification in guideline #1.

a. Periodic reassessment is extremely important, and includes documentation of:

   i. Level of function

   ii. Progress towards predetermined goals

   iii. Presence of adverse events

   iv. Compliance (or lack of)

b. **In patients who are at high risk** or display evidence of aberrant drug-related behaviors, **clinicians should periodically obtain urine drug screens or other information** to confirm compliance to the treatment plan.

c. **In patients not at high risk** or displaying evidence of aberrant drug-related behaviors, clinicians should periodically obtain urine drug screens or other information to confirm compliance to the treatment plan.

"...use of tools with strong content, face and construct validity, such as the PADT and COMM, are recommended as an efficient method of assessment and documentation." It is also stated that urine drug screening is *"likely to result in a higher yield in patients with risk factors for drug abuse or diversion."*

6. **High Risk Patients**

Chronic noncancer pain occurs frequently in patients with either a history of aberrant drug-related behavior, or psychiatric co-morbid history.

a. **High-risk patients should only be treated by clinicians that are able to implement more frequent and stringent monitoring approaches**, such as a mental health or addiction specialist. "In such situations clinicians should strongly consider consultation with a mental health or addiction specialist."

b. Clinicians need to consider that in patients engaged in aberrant drug-related behaviors, **there may be a need for restructuring of therapy**, referral for assistance in management, or discontinuation of opioid therapy.

7. **Dose Escalations, High-Dose Opioid Therapy, Opioid Rotation, and Indications for Discontinuation of Therapy**

Patients that are resistant to relatively high doses of chronic opioids can be quite challenging to manage. In all cases, a cause for dose escalation must be considered to be an indicator of substance abuse or diversion. There is no absolute dose ceiling, but there should always be a theoretical limit to the escalation of the dosing scheme.

a. When repeated escalations are necessary, **potential causes for the increased need**, as well as risks and benefits should be reconsidered.

b. Increased vigilance, such as more frequent follow-up visits, should be considered in patients on high-dose opioid therapy.

c. Opioid rotation should be considered for issues such as tolerance of adverse effects or unsatisfactory efficacy.

d. Discontinuation of opioid therapy is recommended by **tapering or weaning** for patients who repeatedly engage in aberrant drug-related behaviors.

8. Opioid-Related Adverse Effects

While opioids can be quite effective in the treatment of chronic noncancer pain, they also carry a fairly substantial adverse effect profile, with constipation being the most commonly bothersome adverse effect.

a. Common adverse effects, such as constipation, nausea and vomiting, sedation, sexual dysfunction, fatigue, or itching, need to be anticipated and addressed appropriately.

b. Respiratory depression may occur when the opioid doses are high, titrated too rapidly, combined with other medications that may potentiate the effect (such as benzodiazepines), or in patients with other underlying conditions, such as sleep apnea or obesity.

9. Use of Psychotherapeutic Co-interventions

"When pain is accompanied by co-morbidities, impaired function, or psychological disturbances, chronic opioid therapy is likely to be most effective as **part of multimodality treatment** that addresses all of these domains. Clinicians should routinely integrate therapies that target the psychosocial and functional factors that contribute to or are affected by chronic noncancer pain."

- Psychotherapeutic co-interventions, such as **cognitive-behavioral therapy**, along with other interdisciplinary therapy and other adjunctive non-opioid therapies should be routinely integrated into long-term opioid treatment.

10. Driving and Work Safety

Opioids may often cause **drowsiness, decreased concentration, or slower reaction times**, especially at the initiation of treatment. Obviously, these phenomena could impair a patient's ability to drive a vehicle, or operate dangerous machinery. "In the absence of signs or symptoms of impairment, **no evidence exists to suggest that patients maintained on chronic opioid therapy should be restricted from driving or engaging in most work activities**."

- Counseling about transient or lasting cognitive impairment must be addressed with patients.

11. Identifying a Medical Home and When to Obtain Consultation

It has been shown that pain patients do better when they have access to a clinician who coordinates, and provides the majority of their health care needs. The attributes of effective primary care were described recently in a model known as the patient-centered primary care "medical home."

a. A clinician needs to be identified as the person with primary responsibility for the patient's overall medical care. This may or may not be the clinician prescribing the chronic opioid therapy, but should coordinate consultation and all communication among all disciplines involved in the patient's care.

b. Consultation should be considered, as in any other situation, when the treating clinician feels that the patient may benefit from other resources beyond their capability.

12. Breakthrough Pain

Patients on chronic opioid therapy may experience **episodes of increased pain**, or breakthrough pain. This type of pain **needs to be assessed separately** from the baselinepain. Appropriate evaluation may include diagnostic testing, and further investigation.

a. **Additional prn opioids** may be needed for patients on around-the-clock therapy, and should always be used based on a thorough risk-benefit analysis.

b. Vigilance for aberrant drug-related behavior or diversion must always be considered.

13. Opioids in Pregnancy

As in other situations, **clinicians should counsel women of childbearing capacity** about the risks and benefits of chronic opioid therapy during and after pregnancy.

a. In most situations, **use of opioids during pregnancy should be discouraged or minimized**, unless benefits are determined to outweigh the risks.

b. In the event that chronic opioid therapy is utilized during pregnancy, the needs of the mother and the baby need to be appropriately anticipated.

14. Opioid Policies

Surveys show that **clinicians have a poor or limited understanding of the laws**, regulations, and other policies that govern the prescribing, dispensing, or administration of controlled substances, including opioid analgesics.

a **It is imperative that clinicians become aware of local policies** surrounding the medical use of chronic opioids for noncancer pain patients, such as:

   i. Federal laws

   ii. State laws

   iii. Regulatory guidelines

   iv. Policy statements

These guidelines may seem quite simplistic if taken individually. They are significant collectively as a formulated plan to use opioids safely and appropriately in this very important population of patients. Very often, noncancer pain patients are denied the appropriate course of treatment, or quantity of therapeutic agent as the result of what has been a deficit in a strategic plan for approaching the long-term treatment of chronic pain with opioids. These guidelines can do much to improve the quality of care of these patients, and increase comfort levels of clinicians if utilized in their complete form. Coupled with good clinical judgment, these recommendations can provide clinicians with the framework for safer use of opioids and more efficacious care of patients with chronic noncancer pain, minimizing the risk associated with their use[13].

The decision to prescribe opioids for the treatment of pain is no different than the prescribing of any medication for any disorder. As in the example of insulin treatment for diabetes, all therapies have potential complications, which are more likely to occur (by definition) in high-risk patients. Therefore, patients should be screened for risk level on initiation of therapy and reassessed periodically. The **SOAPP**® (**S**creener and **O**pioid **A**ssessment for **P**atients with **P**ain), can be used when considering initiating opioid treatment, and the **COMM**™ (**C**urrent **O**pioid **M**isuse **M**easure) can be used as a follow-up tool for patients who are prescribed opioids. These tools can be downloaded from *www. PainEDU.org*.

If indicated, as mentioned in the above guidelines, opioid therapy can be initiated on a trial basis, and the trial can continue for as long as the patient is on treatment. In general, a trial period of 3 months can be recommended. At each follow-up visit, with a tool such as COMM™, the patient goes through a semi-structured assessment that assesses key outcome variables, but that need not be excessively time-consuming if approached systematically.

Although this chapter is focused on prescribing practices that minimize the risks of opioid therapy, this can be effectively presented in the context of an overall approach to opioid therapy (see Figure 5). Opportunities to optimize outcome, by maximizing efficacy and minimizing risks, present themselves at every point in the algorithm.

■ Figure 5
Algorithm for Opioid Treatment of Chronic Pain

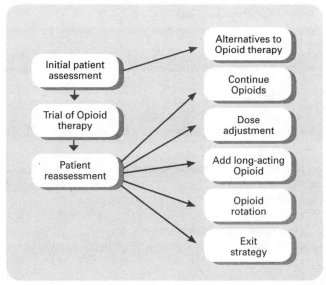

Used with the permission of Nathaniel P. Katz, MD

Initial Patient Pain Assessment

As in all other areas of medicine, the initial assessment of the patient with chronic pain has several purposes, including developing a diagnosis, cataloging previous therapies, understanding the patient's status on multiple dimensions (pain, function, psychological, social), setting treatment goals, and creating a treatment plan. With respect to opioid therapy, the purposes of the initial assessment are to determine whether opioid therapy is indicated, assess previous experience with opioid therapy, and determine the risk of opioid abuse.

The outline below indicates the key elements relevant to opioid therapy that should be added to the routine initial medical evaluation. With these additional elements of the medical history, the clinician can

■ **Table 8.1**
Initial Evaluation Guide

History of present illness (pain)
■ Diagnosis
■ Prior treatments
■ Previous experience with opioid therapy
  • Effectiveness
  • Compliance
  • Subjective experience (e.g., euphoria)
  • Misuse (e.g., for insomnia, stress, mood enhancement)

Past History
■ Illnesses relevant to opioid therapy (e.g., respiratory, hepatic, renal disease)
■ Medical illnesses suggestive of substance abuse
  • Hepatitis
  • Human immunodeficiency virus infection
  • Tuberculosis
  • Cellulitis
  • Sexually transmitted diseases
  • Elevated liver function tests
  • Trauma, burns

Psychiatric History
■ Current or past mental illness
■ History of substance abuse, including alcohol, tobacco
  • None
  • Past, in remission
  • Current
  • Which substances, routes, prescription drugs

Family History
■ Substance abuse
■ Social support system

categorize patients into the following risk strata:

- **Low risk:** *No history of substance abuse; minimal if any risk factors*

  Can be managed by primary care provider

- **Medium risk:** *Past history of substance abuse (no prescription opioid abuse); significant risk factors*

  Can be co-managed with addiction and/or pain specialist specialists

- **High risk:** *Active substance abuse problem; history of prescription opioid abuse*

  Refer patient to center specializing in management of comorbid pain and addictive disorders; opioids may not be appropriate

Initiating an Opioid Trial

If on the basis of the assessment, the patient appears to be an appropriate candidate for opioid therapy, it is appropriate to initiate a trial, as mentioned in the above guidelines. In some situations, many patients are prescribed opioids without a formal declaration of long-term opioid therapy. This occurs, for example, in a patient with chronic pain who receives a short-term opioid prescription for a pain flare and continues to receive frequent refills before the clinician (and patient) realizes that, in fact, the patient is now on long-term opioid therapy. Although in principle these documented steps will be initiated at the time of initiation of opioid therapy, in practice, they are often initiated "when the light bulb goes off."

An important difference between opioid therapy and non-abusable drug therapies is in the role of patient self-report. Some members of the addiction community feel that the patient's self-report in the context of opioid therapy must be taken with a "grain of salt" because in a number of conditions, patient self-report may lose its reliability; this applies to pain intensity, functional improvement, compliance with therapy, and substance abuse–related issues. The clinician accustomed to obeying the mantra of "always believe the patient" must learn to modify this approach in the setting of opioid therapy and to consider self-report as one of many sources of information about the patient's status; this is done for the sake of the patient.

A trial of opioid therapy is usually begun with as-needed doses of a short-acting product combining an opioid and a nonopioid analgesic. Common choices include hydrocodone/acetaminophen, oxycodone/acetaminophen, oxycodone/ibuprofen, and codeine/acetaminophen. The nonopioid component maximizes the balance of analgesia and side effects of the regimen, in an opioid-sparing and synergistic fashion. The use of short-acting as-needed doses allows the clinician and patient to assess the opioid requirement, and allows for relatively more rapid dose adjustments.

Short-acting agents are possibly the most widely abused opioids in the United States. With the exception of extended-release oxycodone products, long-acting products tend to be abused less than short-acting preparations due to the ease with which the extended-release formulation can be converted to a high-potency immediate-release formulation. Also, individuals with addictive disorders tend to be able to comply better with medications that are taken at fixed doses round the clock rather than on an as-needed basis. The patient's pain profile should be taken into account as well: Patients with a fairly consistent pain profile (where pain intensity is more or less the same all the time) may be more likely to succeed with a sustained-release-only regimen; patients with intermittent pain may not do as well. Abuse-deterrent formulations (ADFs) could be potentially effective in supporting opioid access while limiting abuse and its consequences. Several different approaches are being employed including physical barriers to tampering, agonist-antagonist formulations, and alternative methods of administration, all with potential to reduce specific forms of abuse and misuse. See Chapter VI for information about "Abuse-Deterrent Formulations of Opioids."

A final consideration in the choice of opioid is tramadol*. Tramadol is an analgesic that derives part of its pain-relieving properties from an opioid effect (just like morphine), but part from nonopioid effects (inhibition of reuptake of norepinephrine and serotonin, like many ·

---

*The manufacturer of tramadol and the FDA notified health care professionals in May 2010 of changes to the warnings section of the prescribing information for tramadol. The strengthened warning information emphasizes the risk of suicide for patients who are addiction-prone, taking tranquilizers or antidepressant drugs, And also warns of the risk of overdosage .

antidepressants). Tramadol is far less likely to be abused than other opioid analgesics, although it certainly can be abused. Tramadol is now available in an extended-release formulation as well. Patients with insufficient analgesia on tramadol can always be advanced to other opioid therapies. The manufacturer of tramadol and the FDA notified health care professionals in May 2010 of changes to the Warnings section of the prescribing information for tramadol. The strengthened warning information emphasizes the risk of suicide for patients who are addiction-prone, taking tranquilizers or antidepressant drugs, and also warns of the risk of overdosage.

Follow-Up Visit

It is helpful to follow a structured assessment in following patients on long-term opioid therapy. Follow-up assessment that clinicians can use should be based on the "four A's"[14]:

1. **Analgesia:** What is the patient's average pain intensity?
2. **Activities:** How has the patient been functioning?
3. **Adverse events:** Has the patient had side effects?
4. **Aberrant behavior:** Has there been any evidence of abuse, misuse, or addiction?

Based on capturing the above information, the clinician can develop two more "A's": **assessment** and **action** plan.

Analgesia

Patients on opioids for chronic pain rarely enjoy complete pain relief. In fact, many patients live with pain in the "moderate" range—typically 4–7 on a 0–10 numerical rating scale—despite the common perception that opioids are extremely "strong" medications. It is critical to manage patient expectations early so that patients (and clinicians) are not disappointed with the result of partial pain relief and some functional restoration. *In the assessment of analgesia, at least partial pain reduction is necessary evidence for the appropriateness of continuing opioid therapy.* Many clinicians are familiar with the type of patient who, despite ongoing opioid therapy, continues to have reports of severe pain (8–10 out of 10), or even ratings that are "off the scale," but who insist that the opioids are "taking the edge off " the pain. These patients are at high risk for having psychosocial issues amplifying their pain perception, and may constitute an exception to the generally useful dictum that in making decisions about analgesic regimens the clinician should rely primarily on the patient's self-report. Patients with persistently high pain intensity ratings and no evidence of functional improvement should have their dose increased (as long as there are not significant side effects), should have nonopioid analgesic approaches added (medical, rehabilitative, or psychosocial), or should be tapered off opioid therapy.

Activities

A judgment that a patient is indeed benefiting from opioid therapy is more convincing if there has been some evidence of functional improvement. Function can be construed broadly and includes activities of daily living, psychological function, social function, sleep, employment, and so forth. Even a slight improvement in pain intensity accompanied by clear evidence of increased function is very persuasive of opioid benefit. On the other hand, a picture of persistently high pain scores and no functional improvement—or actual functional deterioration—generally suggests that an opioid taper is appropriate.

Adverse Events

Patients have many more adverse effects of opioid therapy than they report. Therefore, adverse effects should be elicited prospectively. Often, patients fear that if they report side effects, the medication will be stopped. Although switching opioids is often the most effective solution for opioid-induced side effects, a number of other approaches can be used to address side effects without changing medications, and can thereby improve the patient's outcome on opioid therapy.

Aberrant Behaviors

Many patients use their medication in a way that would not be condoned, or even anticipated by, their clinicians. *Noncompliance* is ubiquitous in medicine and may be unintentional (e.g., taking the wrong dose by mistake, forgetting a dose), intentional but not related to abuse (e.g., taking an extra oxycodone to help sleep, unauthorized dose escalation for a pain flare), or intentional and related to abuse (e.g. taking extra to get high, faking pain to get opioids, using the medication in an out-of-control manner). The clinician seeing the patient for pain often does not have the luxury that an addiction specialist in an addiction treatment center may have, whose patients all openly acknowledge their problematic drug use. The pain clinician often sees a confusing and subtle pattern of behaviors and must make a judgment as to whether the behaviors represent a pattern potentially indicating abuse, addiction, or criminal behavior, or whether the behaviors can be adequately explained by more benign causes: cognitive or language difficulties, administrative or insurance reasons, comorbid psychological conditions, or pseudoaddiction. Research has shown that most patients engage in a number of aberrant behaviors. The challenge is for the clinician to judge when these aberrant behaviors occur and what actions to take in view of the fact that confirmation can rarely be made with 100% certainty in the pain management setting.

RE-EVALUATION OF AN OPIOID MANAGEMENT PLAN

Based on the assessment, there are five options for how to handle the opioid therapy:

1. **Continue** it without change

2. **Adjust** the dose regimen

3. **Add** a long- or short-acting agent

4. **Rotate** to another opioid

5. **Discontinue** opioid therapy

Other therapeutics can be implemented as a result of the visit, such as instituting nonopioid analgesic approaches (e.g., acupuncture, physical therapy, psychological therapies, nonopioid analgesics, etc.).

Continuation of Opioid Therapy

Continuation of opioid therapy is not a default decision—it is a specific action that is justified by the patient assessment. Patients who have been stable with their dosing, who are benefiting in terms of pain reduction and/or improved function, who are tolerating their medication, and who have minimal aberrant behaviors are appropriate for continuation of therapy. Continuing therapy that is patently ineffective (whether or not it "takes the edge off ") or that has been associated with functional deterioration (not explained by other factors) cannot be justified, whether or not there are other available management options.

Dose Adjustment

The dose can be too high, too low, or not administered optimally. Opioids need to be dosed on a case-by-case basis based on the response. Patients with persistent unrelieved pain, who are otherwise tolerating their dosage, can have their dose increased. Patients with dose-limiting side effects need to have their dose decreased, or their side effects managed another way; the dose cannot be increased. For some patients, the therapeutic index can be improved by altering the mode of administration. For example, patients with side effects at the peak of exposure to a short-acting opioid may do better with smaller, more frequent doses or with a long-acting opioid. In contrast, patients on long-acting opioids with side effects during periods of minimal pain may do better on intermittent doses of a short-acting opioid. Finally, some patients cannot find a dose that allows them to enjoy pain relief without significant side effects. Those patients are candidates for opioid rotation. If a therapeutic index cannot be found with a few opioids for an individual patient, that patient is probably not a candidate for opioid therapy and should be moved to "exit strategy."

Addition of a Long- or Short-Acting Opioid

There is little if any evidence that long-acting opioids are better in general than short-acting opioids for patients with chronic pain. However, there are particular types of patients for whom the addition of a long-acting opioid to a short-acting one, or even the substitution of long-acting for short-acting, may improve clinical outcomes. The clearest example is the patient who is taking substantial doses of short-acting opioids multiple times per day. Because tolerance is often first manifested by decreased duration of action, such patients may be forced to take their medication every 2 or 3 hours. The addition of a long-acting agent may be extremely help-ful. Another example is the patient with a compliance problem, due either to cognitive issues or abuse-related problems. Stopping the short-acting medication and substituting a long-acting medication may allow such patients to continue to benefit from opioid therapy in a manner that reduces risk. It is important for clinicians to realize that all currently marketed opioids can be abused, and substituting a long-acting opioid for a short-acting one may reduce risk in some circumstances but does not eliminate the risk completely. Furthermore, some long-acting opioids, such as extended-release oxycodone, are highly prized by abusers.

Opioid Rotation

It has been observed that individual patients may do poorly on one opioid but better after switching to another. Various explanations have been offered for this phenomenon. One explanation is that because some opioids are associated with the accumulation of toxic metabolites after prolonged use (e.g., morphine, hydromorphone), switching to another allows for the clearance of metabolites accumulated from the first opioid. Another theory is that different opioids may bind in different patterns to subtypes of the opioid receptor, providing different profiles of efficacy and side effects. Regardless, if a patient cannot seem to find an effective and well-tolerated dose of one opioid, it is reasonable to try one or two more opioids before giving up on opioid therapy, or referring to a specialist for further management. It is of critical importance to note that switching patients who are on substantial doses of one opioid to another opioid can be tricky and, if done inappropriately, can lead to underdosing, severe painful flare-ups, withdrawal, or overdose and death, particularly with methadone. Clinicians should have a clear sense of their comfort zone with opioid rotation and should get input as needed.

Exit Strategy

When is it appropriate to stop opioid therapy in an individual patient? Although there has been little guidance on this issue, the following list of criteria is reasonable:

- There has been **no convincing benefit** from opioid therapy despite reasonable attempts at dose adjustment, management of side effects, and opioid rotation.

- Opioids **cannot be tolerated** at a dose that provides meaningful analgesia.

- Persistent **compliance problems** exist despite a patient treatment agreement and efforts at appropriate limit setting.

- Presence of a comorbid condition can make opioid therapy **more likely to harm than help**, such as an active substance abuse problem. (Note that the risk-benefit of opioid therapy depends as much on the treatment setting as on the patient and the medicine.)

**It is critically important to distinguish between abandoning opioid therapy, abandoning pain management, and abandoning the patient.** Exiting a patient from opioid therapy is often difficult for clinicians because of the patient's possible failure to understand that when this decision is made, it is for the welfare of the patient, not for the welfare of the doctor. Approaching the decision to taper off opioid therapy from the perspective of helping the patient helps avoid many (but not all) awkward confrontations. There are many other approaches to pain management than opioid therapy, and a patient can be tapered off from opioid therapy while alternative pain management approaches are pursued (albeit with reasonable expectations). Also, abandoning opioid therapy does not mean abandoning the patient. Often, the most reasonable course is to offer the patient continued medical guidance, even in the case of an addicted patient who pursues co-management of the addictive disorder.

DOCUMENTATION

As in all cases, but especially when treating high-risk patients and those with substance-use disorders, the clinician should keep accurate and complete records. Within the records, the following information should be included:

- The pertinent medical history and physical examination

- Diagnostic, therapeutic, and laboratory results

- Evaluations and consultations

- Mutually understood treatment objectives

- Discussion of risks and benefits (informed consent *and* medication agreement)

- Treatments

- Medications (including date, type, dosage, and quantity prescribed)

- Instructions and agreements

- Periodic reviews of progress, treatment goals, and the medication agreement

Records should remain current and be maintained in an accessible manner and readily available for review.

REFERENCES

1. Swegle JM, Logemann C. Management of common opioid-induced adverse effects. *Am Fam Physician*. 2006 Oct 15; 74(8):1347–1354.

2. Smith H, Bruckenthal P. Implications of opioid analgesia for medically complicated patients. *Drugs Aging*. 2010 May; 27(5):417–33.

3. Tatro DS, ed. *Drug Interaction Facts*. St. Louis, MO: Facts and Comparisons; 2001.

4. Pharmacist's Letter / Prescriber's Letter. January 2008. Volume 24. Number 240106. http://www.harmreduction.org/downloads/Alcohol-Drug%20Interaction%20Chart%20CR07165.pdf. Accessed July 6, 2010.

5. Weatherman R, Crabb DW. Alcohol and medication interactions. *Alcohol Res Health*. 1999; 23:40–54.

6. Joranson D, Gilson AM. Drug crime is a source of abused pain medications in the United States. *J Pain Symptom Manage*. 2005; 30:299–301

7. Katz NP, Adams EH, Chilcoat H. Challenges in the development of prescription opioid abuse-deterrent formulations. *Clin J Pain*. 2007 Oct; 23(8):648–60.

8. Substance Abuse and Mental Health Services Administration, Office of Applied Studies. (June 17, 2010). *The TEDS Report: Changing Substance Abuse Patterns among Older Admissions: 1992 and 2008*. Rockville, MD.

9. Fleming MF, Balousek SL, Klessig CL, Mundt MP, Brown DD. Substance use disorders in a primary care sample receiving daily opioid therapy. *J Pain*. 2007 Jul; 8(7):573–82. Epub 2007 May 11.

10. Federation of State Medical Boards of the United States, Inc. Model policy for the use of controlled substances for the treatment of pain. *J Pain Palliat Care Pharmacother*. 2005; 19(2):73-78.

11. The Comprehensive Drug Abuse Prevention and Control Act of 1970. Pub. L. No. 91–513, 84 Stat. 1236 (Oct 27, 1970).

12. Food and Drug Administration. Risk Evaluation and Mitigation Strategies for Certain Opioid Drugs; Notice of Public Meeting. Docket No. FDA–2009–N–0143. *Federal Register*. Apr 2009; 74(74).

13. Chou R, Fanciullo GJ, Fine PG, et al. Clinical guidelines for the use of chronic opioid therapy in chronic noncancer pain. *The Journal of Pain*. 2009; 10(2):113–130.

14. Passik SD, Kirsh KL, Whitcomb L, et al. A new tool to assess and document pain outcomes in chronic pain patients receiving opioid therapy. *Clin Ther*. 2004 Apr; 26(4):552–561.

Glossary

Abuse. <u>Any</u> use of a legal or illegal medication or substance by intentional self-administration *for a nonmedical purpose*, such as altering one's state of consciousness, e.g., "getting high."

Acupuncture. A procedure in which specific body areas associated with peripheral nerves are pierced with fine needles to produce anesthesia, relieve pain, and promote therapy.

Acute pain. The result of an injury or potential injury to body tissues and activation of nociceptive nerve fibers at the site of local tissue damage. This type of pain is usually time-limited and occurs after trauma, surgery, or a disease process. Acute pain is generally thought to have the biological functions of alerting the individual to harm and preparing for the "fight-or-flight" response to danger.

Addiction. A primary, chronic, neurobiologic disease with genetic, psychosocial, and environmental factors influencing its development and manifestations. Addiction involves a compulsive desire to use a drug despite continued harm.

Adjuvants. Pain relieving medications whose primary indication traditionally is not for the treatment of pain. Adjuvants may be used to treat certain types of pain (e.g. neuropathic pain), or may be used to augment the analgesic effect of opioids or to manage their side effects. This term is derived mainly from the cancer pain literature and includes medications such as tricyclic antidepressants and anticonvulsants that were initially prescribed for other indications.

Algology. The science and study of pain. An algologist is a student, investigator, or practitioner of algology.

Allodynia. The presence of pain from a stimulus that is not normally painful. For example, pain caused by clothing or bedclothes rubbing over the skin would be considered allodynia.

Analgesia. Absence of pain in response to stimulation that would normally be painful.

Anesthesia. Loss of feeling or awareness. A general anesthetic puts the person to sleep. A local anesthetic causes loss of feeling in a part of the body, such as a tooth or an area of skin, without affecting consciousness. Regional anesthesia numbs a larger part of the body such as a leg or arm, also without affecting consciousness. The term "conduction anesthesia" encompasses both local and regional anesthetic techniques.

Anergia. Lack of energy.

Anhedonia. Psychological condition characterized by the inability to derive pleasure from normally enjoyable activities. This is one indication of depression.

Ankylosing spondylitis. A type of arthritis that causes chronic inflammation of the spine and the sacroiliac joints. Chronic inflammation in these areas causes pain and stiffness in and around the spine. Over time, chronic spinal inflammation (spondylitis) can lead to a complete cementing together (fusion) of the vertebrae, a process called ankylosis. Ankylosis causes total loss of mobility of the spine.

Anticonvulsants. Medications used to treat seizures. Due to presumed common mechanisms underlying epilepsy and neuropathic pain, many anticonvulsants are effective in treating neuropathic pain.

Antidepressants. A class of medications used to treat depression that includes tricyclic-type antidepressants (TCAs), selective serotonin reuptake inhibitors (SSRIs), serotonin-noradrenaline reuptake inhibitors (SNRIs), and monoamine oxidase inhibitors (MAOs). Some antidepressants, especially TCAs, have been found to have analgesic efficacy. Antidepressants are often used for treating depression associated with chronic pain conditions. See SSRI, SNRI, and TCA for more information. Other antidepressants in a miscellaneous category are bupropion, mirtazapine, nefazodone, and trazodone.

Anxiety. A feeling of apprehension and fear characterized by physical symptoms, such as palpitations, sweating, and feelings of stress.

Antiemetic. Medication used for nausea and vomiting. Antiemetics are also used to facilitate treatment in migraine headaches that cause vomiting.

Arthritis. A generic term that describes more than 100 different conditions. It is a disorder of a joint where two bones meet, which may be manifested on physical examination by swelling, redness, warmth, or tenderness in the joint, or may be demonstrated on radiograph by loss of the joint space, formation of spurs, erosions, or cysts in the bone.

Arthroplasty. Implantation of a prosthesis in a joint.

Biofeedback. Feedback from a device or computer to provide information about physiological processes about which patients are not normally aware (e.g., muscle tension, skin temperature). Biofeedback may help relieve muscle tension caused by bracing muscles due to chronic pain.

Breakthrough pain. An exacerbation of pain that occurs beyond constant, background pain. Short-acting opioids are often prescribed for this purpose. One subcategory of breakthrough pain is "incident pain," which is pain that is provoked by certain "incidents," e.g. walking.

Cancer pain. Pain associated with cancer, which can be the result of cancer itself or treatments for cancer (e.g. surgery, radiation, chemotherapy). It can be visceral, somatic, or neuropathic in nature.

Capsaicin. A component of certain plants, including cayenne and red pepper, used topically to relieve minor arthritis pain and nerve pain.

Cannabis. The botanical name for the marijuana plant. Its full name is Cannibis sativa. Use of cannabis produces a mild sense of euphoria, as well as impairments in judgment and lengthened response time. Cannabis may be smoked or eaten.

Catastrophizing. A cognitive coping style that involves an increasingly downward cycle of negative thoughts that has been associated with depression and negative outcomes in chronic pain.

Causalgia. A syndrome of sustained burning pain, allodynia, and hyperpathia after a traumatic nerve lesion, often combined with vasomotor and sudomotor (relating to the nerves that stimulate the sweat glands to activity) dysfunction, and later trophic changes.

Central Pain. Pain initiated or caused by a primary lesion or dysfunction in the central nervous system.

Central sensitization. Process by which pain is amplified and maintained centrally (in the spinal cord or brain), in addition to the processes in peripheral tissues. This general concept is thought to underlie some types of allodynia or hyperalgesia. It may also explain why surgically removing the "cause of the pain" may not eliminate the pain.

Centralization. This is a loosely defined term of a pain process that begins in the periphery and over time becomes sustained partially or completely by central mechanisms. This concept overlaps with that of central sensitization. Centralization or central sensitization may also underlie evolution of the phenomenology of a chronic pain syndrome, such as the "spread" of reflex sympathetic dystrophy to other limbs.

Chiropractic. A system of diagnosis and treatment based on the concept that the nervous system coordinates all of the body's functions, and that disease results from a lack of normal nerve function. Chiropractic employs manipulation and adjustment of body structures, such as the spinal column, so that pressure on nerves coming from the spinal cord due to displacement (subluxation) of a vertebral body may be relieved.

Chronic pain. Pain that persists beyond the expected healing period. Chronic pain may be associated with levels of underlying pathology that do not explain the presence or extent of pain, and is often associated with affective and behavioral responses to the chronicity of the pain. Sources often define chronic pain as that persisting beyond three or six months after an injury.

Cluster headaches. A strictly unilateral headache, usually occurring once or a few times a day at a characteristic time (e.g. 1a.m.), lasting for 15–180 minutes, occurring in a series which lasts for weeks to months, separated by remissions lasting from months to years. Cluster headaches are usually episodic, but have been known to last up to 14 days. Cluster headaches tend to occur more often in men, usually are unilateral, but can shift from side to side in some patients.

Cognitions. Thoughts that can exert powerful effects on physical reactions, as well as responses to and interpretations of pain on the patient.

Cognitive-behavioral therapy. A form of psychological treatment that combines cognitive psychotherapeutic techniques with behavioral techniques and is used to help patients change their thoughts and behaviors to better cope with pain, decrease negative affect and increase functioning.

Complementary and Alternative Medicine (CAM). Approaches to medical treatment that are outside of mainstream medical training. Complementary medicine treatments used for pain include: acupuncture, low-level laser therapy, meditation, aroma therapy, Chinese medicine, dance therapy, music therapy, massage, herbalism, therapeutic touch, yoga, osteopathy, chiropractic treatments, naturopathy, and homeopathy.

Conscious sedation. Light sedation during which the patient retains airway reflexes and responses to verbal stimuli.

Constipation. A condition in which bowel movements are infrequent or incomplete.

CRPS type I (RSD). Chronic pain that includes clinical findings of regional pain, sensory changes, allodynia, abnormalities of temperature, abnormal pseudomotor activity, edema, and an abnormal skin color. These findings may occur after a noxious event.

CRPS type II (Causalgia). Includes all the features of CRPS I, as well as a peripheral nerve lesion.

Cryotherapy. The therapeutic use of cold to reduce discomfort, limit progression of tissue edema, or break a cycle of muscle spasm.

Cyclooxygenase. Refers to a particular enzyme involved in the formation of prostaglandins in the body. The enzyme may be important in the natural physiology in a particular organ or cell, or may be involved in the formation of prostaglandins that induce inflammation in a joint, in which case it may be detrimental.

Cyclooxygenase-1 (COX-1). An enzyme that is normally present in the body for physiologic reasons. It is also called constitutive cyclooxygenase, COX-1 is produced physiologically in the stomach and protects the lining of the stomach.

Cyclooxygenase-2 (COX-2). The inducible form of cyclooxygenase that arises with joint inflammation and is involved in the diseases of the joints. COX-2 is produced in the joint when induced by inflammation.

Deafferentation Pain. Pain due to loss of sensory input into the central nervous system (as can occur with avulsion of the brachial plexus), or other types of peripheral nerve lesions. Can also be due to pathologic lesions of the central nervous system.

Delirium. A syndrome characterized by combinations of cognitive deficits, fluctuating levels of consciousness, changes in sleep patterns, psychomotor agitation, hallucinations, delusions and/or perceptual abnormalities. Causes are multifactorial and can include psychotropic medications, opioids, metabolic changes, cancer treatment, sepsis, brain tumor, or metastases.

Depression. An illness characterized by a low mood that impairs normal functioning for a prolonged period of time. May be accompanied by loss of pleasure in usual activities, loss of appetite, poor sleep, agitation, fatigue, feelings of worthlessness, difficulty concentrating, suicidal thoughts.

Dermatome. A sensory segment of the skin supplied by a specific nerve root.

Diabetic neuropathy. Damage or dysfunction of the peripheral nervous system due to diabetes mellitus. There are several distinct subtypes of diabetic neuropathy, each with different clinical features, prognosis, and treatment approaches. These include diabetic third cranial nerve palsy, diabetic radiculopathy, diabetic amyotrophy (radiculo-plexopathy), and peripheral polyneuropathy (the classic "stocking-and-glove neuropathy."). Also see painful peripheral polyneuropathy.

Disc. Shortened terminology for an intervertebral disc, a disk-shaped piece of specialized tissue that separates the bones of the spinal column.

Distraction. A cognitive coping technique that involves turning attention away from painful sensations.

Diversion. The intentional removal of a medication from legitimate distribution and dispensing channels.

Dysesthesia. An unpleasant abnormal sensation, whether spontaneous or evoked. **Note:** Compare with pain and with paresthesia. Special cases of dysesthesia include hyperalgesia and allodynia. A dysesthesia should always be unpleasant and a paresthesia should not be unpleasant, although it is recognized that the borderline may present some difficulties when it comes to deciding as to whether a sensation is pleasant or unpleasant. It should always be specified whether the sensations are spontaneous or evoked.

Dyspareunia. Painful or difficult coitus.

Dysphoria. An emotional state marked by anxiety, depression, and restlessness.

Epidural. Situated within the spinal canal, on or outside the dura mater (the tough membrane surrounding the spinal cord); synonyms are extradural and peridural.

Equianalgesic dose. The dose of one opioid that gives the same amount of pain relief as a dose of another opioid, or another route of administration. For example, the equianalgesic dose of hydromorphone, for 10 mg of IM morphine, is 1.5 mg IM. These comparisons are always averages, and vary from patient to patient.

Facet Joint. The facet joints are small joints that are located on the back of the spine, one on each side. Each vertebra is connected by facet joints. They provide stability to the spine by interlocking two vertebrae.

Fibromyalgia syndrome (FMS). A common chronic, widespread pain syndrome characterized by a set of well-defined symptoms. Etiologic or pathologic findings are not established.

Goniometer. An instrument for measuring angles (as of a joint).

Gout. Condition characterized by abnormally elevated levels of uric acid in the blood, recurring attacks of joint inflammation (arthritis), deposits of hard lumps of uric acid in and around the joints.

Full or pure opioid agonists. Class of opioids that produce analgesic effects by binding to the mu-opioid receptor. Opioid analgesics do not have a ceiling effect for analgesia and do not interfere with the effects of other opioids in this class when prescribed simultaneously. Examples include morphine, fentanyl, oxycodone, oxymorphone, hydromorphone, meperidine, codeine, and methadone. They are distinguished from the partial agonists, agonist/antagonists, and pure antagonists.

Heat. Refers to the application of heat via hot packs, hot water bottles, moist compresses, heating pads, chemical and gel packs, and immersion in water for the purpose of relief of pain.

Herniated disc. Rupturing of the tissue that separates the vertebral bones of the spinal column.

Herpes Zoster. Also called shingles, zona, and zoster. The culprit is the varicella-zoster virus. Primary infection with this virus causes chickenpox (varicella). At this time the virus infects nerves (namely, the dorsal root ganglia) where it remains latent (lies low) for years. It can then be reactivated to cause shingles with blisters over the distribution of the affected nerve, often accompanied by intense pain and itching.

Hospice. A special way of caring for people with terminal illnesses and their families by meeting the patient's physical, emotional, social, and spiritual needs, as well as the needs of the family. The goals of hospice are to keep the patient as comfortable as possible by relieving pain and other symptoms; to prepare for a death that follows the wishes and needs of the patient; and to reassure both the patient and family members by helping them to understand and manage what is happening.

Hyperalgesia. The phenomenon whereby stimuli that are normally painful produce exaggerated pain. It can be ascertained by the response to single and multiple pinpricks on neurologic examination.

Hyperesthesia. Increased sensitivity to stimulation, excluding the special senses. **Note:** The stimulus and locus should be specified. Hyperesthesia may refer to various modes of cutaneous sensibility, including touch and thermal sensation without pain, as well as to pain. The word is used to indicate both diminished threshold to any stimulus and an increased response to stimuli that are normally recognized. Allodynia is suggested for pain after stimulation that is not normally painful. Hyperesthesia includes both allodynia and hyperalgesia, but the more specific terms should be used wherever they are applicable.

Hyperpathia. A painful syndrome characterized by increased reaction to a stimulus, especially a repetitive stimulus, as well as increased threshold.

Hypnosis. A state of heightened awareness and focused concentration that can be used to manipulate the perception of pain.

Hypoesthesia. Decreased sensitivity to stimulation, excluding the special senses. **Note:** Stimulation and locus to be specified.

Hypopathia. Refers to decreased responses to stimulation.

Iatrogenic. Denoting response to medical or surgical treatment induced by treatment itself *(usually used for unfavorable responses)*.

Imagery. A cognitive-behavioral strategy that uses mental images produced by memory or imagination for relaxation or for distraction, depending on the content of the imagery.

Incident pain. Refers to the subset of breakthrough pain that is provoked by specific types of activity (e.g., walking, moving the arm).

Informed Consent. The process of making decisions about medical care that are based on open, honest communication between the health care provider and the patient and/or the patient's family members.

Intrathecal. The area that lies between the arachnoid membrane and pia mater and contains the cerebral spinal fluid (CSF). This subarachnoid space is commonly known as the space where spinal taps are performed.

Lancinating. Characterized by piercing or stabbing sensations.

Long-acting opioids. An opioid with a relatively long duration of action. By tradition, opioids that last longer than about six to eight hours are referred to as long-acting, but the border between short- and long-acting is not precise.

Malingering. Intentional production of false or grossly exaggerated physical or psychological symptoms for the purpose of tangible external incentives, such as obtaining financial compensation, evading criminal prosecution, avoiding work or military duty, and obtaining drugs.

Massage. The manipulation of muscle and connective tissue to enhance the function of those tissues and promote relaxation and well-being. Therapeutic massage can ease tension and reduce pain.

Metabolite accumulation syndrome. Several opioids are metabolized to compounds that can accumulate and produce a characteristic syndrome. The features of this syndrome include anxiety, jitteriness, tremor, multifocal myoclonus, encephalopathy, convulsions, and death. This syndrome classically occurs with normeperidine, a metabolite of meperidine, but has also been reported with morphine and hydromorphone. Other opioids have been reported to cause delirium and similar symptoms, but not due to metabolite accumulation, and without the other characteristic features noted above.

Misuse. Use of a medication (*for a medical purpose*) other than as directed or as indicated, whether willful or unintentional, and whether harm results or not.

Mixed agonists/antagonists. Opioids that block opioid analgesia at the mu-opioid receptor (mu), or are neutral at this receptor while simultaneously producing analgesia by activating the kappa receptor. Available agonist/

antagonists include nalbuphine (Nubain), pentazocine (Talwin), and butorphanol (Stadol).

Modulation. The process of modification of nociceptive signals that takes place in the dorsal horn of the spinal cord and elsewhere with input from ascending and descending pathways.

Morphine conversion guide. A written guideline for the equianalgesic dosing of opioids.

Mu(μ) agonist. Type of opioid; relieves pain by binding to the μ receptor sites in the nervous system.

Multimodal treatment. Treatment by more than one modality (i.e., physical therapy, medical, psychological).

Mucositis. Inflammation or sloughing of the oropharyngeal and gastrointestinal mucosae. This occurs stereotypically after bone marrow transplant and its related chemotherapy, and is a well-recognized stereotypic severe pain syndrome.

Muscle de-education. Occurs when pain or avoiding pain leads to the failure to activate muscles or the abnormal activation of muscles in movement.

Myofascial pain. Pain localized to a region of muscle or soft tissue, associated with *trigger points* (palpable tender nodules or cords within the muscle). By definition the pain must be reproduced by palpation of the trigger point, often with a referred component. The pain may be associated with subjective feelings of "numbness" or "heaviness," but no neurologic deficits. See also trigger points.

Nerve ablation. Surgical or interventional procedures performed on peripheral nerves, the spinal cord, the brain, or brain stem that relieve pain by permanent disruption of nerve pathways.

Nerve block. Infiltration of a local anesthetic around a peripheral nerve so as to produce anesthesia in the area supplied by the nerve.

Neuralgia. Pain in the distribution of a nerve or nerves. **Note:** Common usage, especially in Europe, often implies a paroxysmal quality, but neuralgia should not be reserved for paroxysmal pains.

Neurotransmitter. A chemical that is released from a nerve cell, which thereby transmits an impulse from a nerve cell to another nerve, muscle, organ, or other tissue. A neurotransmitter is a messenger of neurologic information from one cell to another.

Neuritis. Inflammation of a nerve or nerves. **Note:** Not to be used unless inflammation is thought to be present.

Neurogenic pain. Pain initiated or caused by a primary lesion, dysfunction, or transitory perturbation in the peripheral or central nervous system.

Neurolytic block. The injection of a chemical agent to cause destruction and consequent prolonged interruption of peripheral somatic or sympathetic nerves, or in some cases, the neuraxis.

Neuropathic pain. Pain initiated or caused by a primary lesion or dysfunction in the nervous system. **Note:** See also Neurogenic Pain and Central Pain. Peripheral neuropathic pain occurs when the lesion or dysfunction affects the peripheral nervous system. Central pain may be retained as the term when the lesion or dysfunction affects the central nervous system.

Neuropathy. A disturbance of function or pathological change in a nerve: in one nerve, mononeuropathy; in several nerves, mononeuropathy multiplex; if diffuse and bilateral, polyneuropathy. **Note:** Neuritis (q.v.) is a special case of neuropathy and is now reserved for inflammatory processes affecting nerves. Neuropathy is not intended to cover cases like neurapraxia, neurotmesis, section of a nerve, or transitory impact (e.g. a blow, stretching, or an epileptic discharge). The term neurogenic applies to pain due to such temporary perturbations.

Nociceptive pain. Pain that results from injury to or inflammation of somatic tissues.

Nociceptor. A receptor preferentially sensitive to a noxious stimulus or to a stimulus that would become noxious if prolonged.

Nonpharmacologic treatment. Treatment that does not involve use of drugs (e.g., physical therapy, biofeedback, psychological treatment).

Nonsteroidal anti-inflammatory drug (NSAID). Aspirin-like medication that reduces inflammation (and hence pain) arising from injured tissue. *COX-2 selective NSAID:* An NSAID that inhibits the COX-2 isoform of cyclooxygenase, but not the COX-1 form. *Nonselective NSAID:* An NSAID that inhibits both COX-1 and COX-2 isoforms of cyclooxygenase.

Noxious Stimulus. A noxious stimulus is one that is damaging to normal tissues.

Numerical Rating Scale (NRS). A method of rating pain intensity that involves written or verbal numerical notation of pain (e.g., 11-point scale from 0 "no pain" to 10 "worst possible pain").

Opiate receptor. Opiate-binding sites found throughout primary afferents and the neuraxis.

Opioid. A morphine-like medication that produces pain relief. The term opioid is preferred to the term narcotic; it refers to natural, semi-synthetic, and synthetic medications that relieve pain by binding to opioid receptors in the nervous system. Opioid is also preferred to the term opiate because it includes all agonists and antagonists with morphine-like activity, as well as naturally occurring and synthetic opioid peptides.

Osteoarthritis (OA). A disease of the cartilage that progressively produces a local tissue response, mechanical change, and failure of function. The disease typically affects weight-bearing joints asymmetrically. It is the most common form of arthritis.

Pain. An unpleasant sensory and emotional experience associated with actual or potential tissue damage, or described in terms of such damage.

Pain assessment. Evaluation of a variety of aspects of perceived sensations of pain, including intensity, duration, frequency, description, location, and emotional responses.

Pain behaviors. Verbal or nonverbal expressions including behavioral reactions, such as grimacing, rubbing the affected part, guarding, restricting movement, and sighing.

Pain threshold. The least experience of pain that a subject can recognize as pain.

Pain tolerance level. The greatest level of pain that a subject is prepared to tolerate.

Painful peripheral polyneuropathy. A generalized disorder of peripheral nerves, usually affecting the distal fibers, with proximal shading, typically occurring symmetrically. They may be classified as axonal or demyelinating and have many causes, particularly metabolic and toxic. Diabetic, alcoholic, vasculitic, and idiopathic tend to be the most painful types.

Palliative care. The total care of patients with progressive, incurable illness. In palliative care, the focus of care is on quality of life. Control of pain and other physical symptoms, and psychological, social, and spiritual problems, are the most important aspects of palliative care.

Paresthesia. An abnormal sensation, whether spontaneous or evoked. Note: Compare with dysesthesia.

Partial agonists. Opioid analgesics that produce analgesia by binding to the mu opioid receptor, but with less intrinsic efficacy at that receptor than "full agonists." These agents have a ceiling effect for analgesia and may precipitate withdrawal if administered to a physically dependent patient. Examples of partial agonists include nalbuphine, pentazocine, and butorphanol.

Patient-controlled analgesia (PCA). Analgesics self-administered by a patient who has received instruction in doing so; usually refers to self-dosing with an intravenous, subcutaneous, epidural, or intrathecal opioid (e.g., morphine) administered by means of a programmable pump.

Pathophysiology. The physiology of abnormal states.

Peripheral neurogenic pain. Pain initiated or caused by a primary lesion or dysfunction or transitory perturbation in the peripheral nervous system.

Peripheral neuropathic pain. Pain initiated or caused by a primary lesion or dysfunction in the peripheral nervous system.

Peripheral sensitization. Process by which neurons in peripheral nerves become abnormally responsive to noxious or non-noxious stimuli, thereby facilitating exaggerated pain perception.

Perception. The final process by which the subject integrates all nociceptive and modulating influences, in the context of psychological and social background and situation information, to form the final experience of pain.

Phantom pain. Pain that develops after an amputation. To the patient, the pain feels like it is coming from the missing body part.

Pharmacotherapy. The treatment of diseases and symptoms with medications.

Physical dependence. A state of adaptation that is manifested by a drug class specific withdrawal syndrome that can be produced by abrupt cessation, rapid dose reduction, decreasing blood level of the drug, or administration of an antagonist.

Physical modalities. Physical methods such as heat, cold, massage, or exercise to relieve pain.

Physical therapy. Physical interventions, including passive modalities (i.e., application of heat and cold) and active modalities (e.g., range of motion, exercise) used to strengthen muscles, increase cardiovascular activity, and restore normal functioning.

Postherpetic neuralgia (PHN). Pain persisting beyond the healing of an acute herpes zoster rash. More recently, PHN has been redefined by some as zoster-associated pain, recognizing that this is a spectrum of pain that occurs before, during, and for variable times after acute herpes zoster.

Primary afferent nociceptors. Pain receptors (A-delta or C-fibers) that respond to noxious mechanical, thermal, and chemical stimuli.

Primary headaches. Headaches that are autonomous without a specific lesion or disease process.

Progressive muscle relaxation. A cognitive-behavioral strategy in which muscles are alternately tensed and then relaxed in a systematic fashion.

Pseudoaddiction. Is a term that is used to describe behavior that appears like addictive, "drug- seeking" behavior, but is actually an effort to obtain pain relief. Behaviors from pseudoaddiction are said to be distinguished from addictive behaviors when the behaviors resolve after treatment of pain.

Psychiatric comorbidities. Concomitant psychiatric disorders that occur in individuals with a medical condition such as chronic pain.

Psychological approaches. Techniques used to help patients cope with over their pain and deal with emotional factors that can increase pain. Such strategies include biofeedback, imagery, hypnosis, relaxation training, stress management, cognitive-behavioral therapy, and family counseling.

Psychosocial intervention. A therapeutic intervention that uses cognitive, cognitive-behavioral, behavioral, and supportive interventions to relieve pain. These include patient education, interventions aimed at aiding relaxation, psychotherapy, and structured or peer support.

Quantitative sensory testing (QST). Testing of sensations with calibrated stimuli such that both stimulus and response can be quantitated. In common usage, QST refers to the use of devices that apply calibrated thermal (hot or cold) stimuli to the skin in order to record the patient's perception of thermal sensory and pain thresholds.

Radiculopathy. Any disease of the spinal nerve roots and spinal nerves. It is synonymous with radiculitis.

Referred pain. The perception of pain in parts of the body distant from the pathology from which the pain originates. Examples include arm pain during an acute myocardial infarction, or eye pain during vertebral artery dissection.

Refractory pain. Pain that is resistant to ordinary treatment.

Relaxation methods. A variety of techniques to help decrease anxiety and muscle tension; these may include imagery, distraction, and progressive muscle relaxation.

Rescue dose. A bolus or extra dose of medication given as needed (prn) to relieve pain that breaks through despite a regimen of medication that is given at regularly scheduled intervals.

Rest pain. Pain experienced while in an inactive or resting state.

Rheumatoid arthritis (RA). A chronic inflammatory condition in which the body's immune system attacks cartilage, bone, and sometimes internal organs, usually causing joint disease. Joints become inflamed, which leads to swelling, pain, stiffness, and the possible loss of function. It is characterized by a symmetrical pattern of synovitis of the joints leading to progressive destruction.

Sciatica. Pain resulting from irritation of the sciatic nerve, typically felt from the low back to behind the thigh and radiating down below the knee. While sciatica can result from a herniated disc directly pressing on the nerve, any cause of irritation or inflammation of this nerve can reproduce the painful symptoms of sciatica.

Scoliosis. Lateral curvature of the spine.

Secondary headaches. Headache associated with primary disease processes, such as brain tumors, head trauma, vascular disorders, and substance use and withdrawal.

Sensation. In medicine and physiology, sensation refers to the registration of an incoming (afferent) nerve impulse in that part of the brain called the sensorium, which is capable of such perception; therefore, the awareness of a stimulus as a result of its perception by sensory receptors.

Silent nociceptors. Afferent nerves that do not respond to external stimulation unless inflammatory mediators are present.

SNRIs. Serotonin-norepinehrine reuptake inhibitors are a type of antidepressant that acts on different mechanisms than other type of antidepressants. An example is venlafaxine. SNRI-type drugs are generally used to treat depression associated with chronic pain.

Somatoform disorder. Pain that is produced or amplified by psychological processes. Criteria are less restrictive than somatization disorder and require one or more physical complaints that cannot be explained by a general medical condition and cause significant social or occupational distress.

Somatic pain. Pain arising from somatic structures (e.g., skin, bones, muscle, joint). It is typically well-localized ("my left finger"), and worsened by palpation or movement of the affected part.

Somatization disorder. Psychological disorder characterized by a pattern of multiple physical complaints (e.g., pain symptoms, gastrointestinal symptoms, sexual problems), present before the age of 30, which causes significant social and occupational impairment.

Somatosensory. Pertaining to sensations received from all tissues of the body (skin, muscles, joints and viscera).

Spinal stenosis. Narrowing of the spaces in the spine, resulting in compression of the nerve roots or spinal cord by bony spurs or soft tissues, such as discs, in the spinal canal.

Spondylolisthesis. Forward movement of one of the vertebrae in relation to an adjacent vertebra.

SSRIs. Selective serotonin reuptake inhibitors are a type of antidepressant that are generally used to treat depression. Little evidence exists for the analgesic effects of SSRIs. Examples of medications in this class are citalopram, fluoxetine, fluvoxamine, paroxetine, and sertraline.

Stress. A response to a situation that is perceived as threatening.

Stress management. Techniques designed to aid in the reduction of physiologic hyperarousal due to stress.

Substance P. A short chain polypeptide that functions as a neurotransmitter, especially in the transmission of pain impulses from peripheral receptors to the central nervous system.

TENS. Transcutaneous Electrical Nerve Stimulation is a pain reduction technique that involves applying low-voltage electrical stimulation to the skin, putatively stimulating large nerve fibers.

Titration to relief. A gradual increase in pain medication until the highest pain relief is obtained, making the pain as tolerable as possible while minimizing short- and long-term negative effects.

Tolerance. The loss of effect of a pharmacological agent over a prolonged period of use, or the need to escalate the dose of the agent in order to maintain the same pharmacological effect.

Topical analgesics. Analgesics that are applied to the skin or mucosa and act locally, presumably with insignificant systemic exposure. Examples include EMLA cream and the lidocaine patch.

Transdermal analgesics. Analgesics that are applied to the skin or mucosa are systemically absorbed, and produce their therapeutic effects and side effects by systemic actions. Examples include the fentanyl patch and the buprenorphine patch.

Transduction. Process by which noxious stimulation of tissues is translated into neural signals in nociceptive nerve fibers. The deepest understanding of this process relates to the role of endogenous chemicals at afferent nerve endings in translating these stimuli (e.g., a burn) into nociceptive impulses.

Transmission. The process by which nerve signals from the periphery are sent to the dorsal horn of the spinal cord along the nociceptive afferents.

Tricyclic antidepressants. A class of antidepressant that is used clinically for treatment of neuropathic pain and for sleep disturbance, generally in lower doses than required for treating depression. Examples are amitriptyline, doxepin, imipramine, and nortriptyline.

Trigeminal neuralgia. A disorder of the trigeminal nerve that causes brief attacks of severe pain in the lips, cheeks, gums, or chin on one side of the face.

Trigger points. Tender nodules or cords within a muscle, palpation of which reproduces localized and/or radiating pain. Trigger points define *myofascial pain*. This phenomenon is distinct from *tender points*, which are tender areas of muscle or soft tissue *not associated* with palpable abnormalities in the texture of the muscle. Tender points occur in fibromyalgia and rheumatic diseases. See also *myofascial pain*.

Visceral pain. Refers to pain arising from pathology of the visceral organs, such as bowel obstruction or pancreatitis. Such pain is typically poorly localized (e.g., my whole belly hurts) and is associated with visceral symptoms (e.g., nausea, vomiting).

Viscosupplementation. A procedure currently approved for use in osteoarthritis in which viscous fluid is injected into a joint (currently the knee joint), which results in decreased pain and increased mobility.

Visual Analogue Scale (VAS). A method of measuring pain intensity that consists of a 10 cm. line with anchors at the ends. Common anchors are "no pain" and "worst possible pain." Patients draw a vertical line through the horizontal line and the result in centimeters is multiplied by 10, yielding a number between 0 and 100.

Windup. A process that has been observed in experimental animals whereby repeated stimulation of a peripheral structure (e.g. the skin) with an electric or other stimulus produces a greater and greater central response (e.g. pain). The mechanism of windup is thought to be sensitization of neurons in the spinal cord that receive nociceptive input, with the result that subsequent stimuli produce greater effects. Windup is an example of central sensitization, which is in turn an example of neural plasticity.

World Health Organization (WHO) analgesic ladder. Recommendations from the WHO for titration of therapy for cancer pain, referred to as the "analgesic ladder." The ladder presents a three-step algorithm for using medications initially in the treatment of cancer pain, and includes five major treatment concepts: (1) by the mouth, (2) by the clock, (3) by the ladder, (4) for the individual, and (5) with attention to detail.

Index

Page numbers followed by *t* indicate tables; those followed by *f* indicate figures